M000107583

Holistic

22 Expert Holistic Practitioners Help You Heal Mind, Body And Spirit In New Ways

Compiled by Kyra Schaefer

Holistic: 22 Expert Holistic Practitioners Help You Heal Mind, Body And Spirit In New Ways

Copyright © 2019. All rights reserved. Each author in this book retains the copyright to their individual section. Their submissions are printed herein with their permission. Each author is responsible for their individual opinions expressed through their words. No part of this publication may be reproduced, distributed, or transmitted to any form or by any means, including photocopying, recording, or other electronic mechanical methods, without the prior written permission of the publisher.

As You Wish Publishing, LLC Kyra@asyouwishpublishing.com 602-592-1141

ISBN-13: 978-1-951131-93-7

ISBN-10: 1-951131-93-2

Library of Congress Control Number: 2019915851

Compiled by Kyra Schaefer

Edited by Todd Schaefer and Karen Oschmann

Printed in the United States of America.

Nothing in this book or any affiliations with this book is a substitute for medical or psychological help. If you are needing help please seek it.

Dedication

To those wishing to empower their healing abilities

TABLE OF CONTENTS

Foreword by Kyra Schaefer

I was a Clinical Hypnotherapist for 15 years before switching to publishing books that help. I have seen first-hand the power of holistic mental and physical medicine on patients as well as myself. I struggled since childhood with a panic disorder perpetuated by physical and emotional abuse in multiple areas of my life. I had to hit rock bottom to try a different approach to healing. Maybe that is where you are right now? Experts in the Holistic Health field are here to help you as your practitioner.

It took me years of struggling with my anxiety before I finally had the push to make a complete change in my diet, addictions and self-talk that was destroying my life. After suffering a traumatic life-defining event where my ex-fiancé severely beat me, I knew I had to make a change. I was able to hunt down a person who would soon become my mentor in the holistic healing community. Keep in mind this was 20 years ago, anything outside of the mainstream ways of healing were completely taboo, considered dangerous and cultish. When you are in pain for as long as I was in pain, I welcomed taboo and woo-woo with open arms. I had some wild experiences in that environment and I learned to love myself with all these amazing kooky people who were healing the masses. I eventually went to work at the healing center and learned a ton. I emmersed myself into every aspect of healing. However, I felt something was missing. Eventually, I moved and opened my practice and would find the piece to the puzzle I was missing. I took my hypnosis training from Bennett Steller University which is where I was able to heal my anxiety. I learned the tools, and I made it my mission to heal the world of anxiety. You may have guessed, I didn't heal the world. But I did help the thousands of people who would eventually come to my office in Phoenix, AZ. I want you to keep in mind this was a journey that spand several years. My self-healing didn't happen all at once.

One session, one book, one kindness may not heal every discomfort or ailment you have, but it's a step in the right direction. It took many practitioners, many sessions to help me heal and I'm still on my journey. I had to learn to love myself better and heal the places where I betrayed myself physically and mentally which takes time and patience. Especially as I age, my body and mind are different then what they were, and I am easing into all the transitions of my life experience in a holistic way. I didn't do that with the first 40 years of my life because the awareness of all the possibilities wasn't available, now the world is changing, we are aware and getting clearer all the time. I have seen people struggle needlessly, the way I did and my heart goes out to them, which is why we brought these experts together in this book.

Every author in this book has worked with clients through their various modalities and tools. They have helped to create change in the lives of others. In this book your holistic practitioner will share their journey, offer wisdom and insights, as well as, sound results-based approaches to personal wellness you may have not yet tried. I had to hunt down my teachers and experts; with this book, they are all right at your fingertips. You even have their contact information if you would like to reach out to them for a consult.

How to use this book:

Trust your instincts and know you are on the right path. By simply picking up this book, you know there is some area that needs improvement in your life. You may flip to any page or chapter randomly, and the insight will flow to your current question. You may also go to any section and do its exercises. You will get to know the authors as they express their journey and how they came to this place in their lives that has caused them to take a leap of faith and offer encouragement to others.

However, you choose to use this book, please know you are never alone in your endeavors. We have all been through something in our lives that have caused us to question or doubt ourselves, and now we have a resource we can turn to and create more possibility, more positivity and more integrity in our health and healing process.

Thank you for taking the time to absorb the vast years of combined knowledge in this book. I can't begin to tell you how honored I am to be in the presence of such amazing people. They have made a difference in my life, and I hope that you gain new awareness in yours as well.

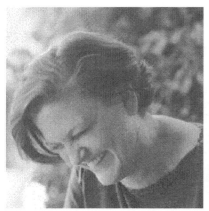

Kyra Schaefer, founder of the independent publishing company, As You Wish Publishing, a business dedicated to making book publishing accessible for aspiring authors who want to publish solo books and participate in collaborative books. Kyra helps authors get their messages heard to bring hope-filled, real-life stories to the world. Her passion is to debunk the myth that writing is difficult and only available for a lucky chosen few.

CHAPTER

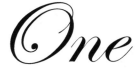

Generational Healing
By Ana Evans

ANA EVANS

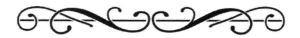

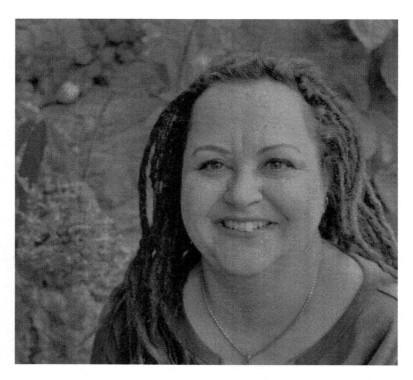

It has been said that to understand something, you must stand under its authority, allowing yourself to experience it. Few people understand the concept of a wounded healer like Ana Evans. By a tapestry of 'the right people at the right time,' Ana has journeyed from victim to survivor to thriver. Now, her story is one of a healer. Over time, her unique experience had afforded opportunities to serve in a variety of capacities with various organizations that work with victims of trauma.

Throughout her journey, one thing has become clear: life is not lived fully unless we are helping others find the path to whole, sustainable healing. She believes that story is an integral part of that process and continues to share her story with as many as have ears to hear it. www.givegreatness.com

Acknowledgments

Angel Salathe (1972-2018)—Thank you for being my loving, hard-assed, beautiful teacher. Desiree Hooston and Benny Evans—My babies! Thank you for every challenge. For all the ways you taught me to be a better parent and person. I love you both to the moon and back! Ben Evans Jr.—Thank you for being a good man. Thank you for pursuing your healing in such a beautiful and graceful way. Nicole Piotraschke—Thank you for your support, love, and undying dedication to me getting the words which need to be written, written.

Generational Healing
By Ana Evans

ho·lis·tic (/hōˈlistik/), *adjective*

1. Philosophy: characterized by comprehension of the parts of something as intimately interconnected and explicable only by reference to the whole.

2. Medicine: characterized by the treatment of the whole person, taking into account mental and social factors, rather than only the symptoms of a disease.

True healing is possible when we treat the whole person. True healing only became possible for me when I was willing to look at my whole person. It took a crisis of faith, and of mental, physical, and emotional health to open myself to even begin to look at alternative healing practices.

I carried an enormous amount of trauma that began when I was a young girl. I had participated in almost every modality of therapy that western medicine had to offer. It helped, to an extent. I felt better, and I was able to manage the symptoms of my trauma. Yet, I still carried it like a warm stone in my belly. I wasn't always in a state of panic and anxiety, but it took a lot of work to hold it all at bay. I could function well enough with the weight of it. I wanted better than well enough, though; I wanted to be well. I didn't know what options were available to me outside of western therapy and medicine.

I was busy surviving life. It's strange to say that I was surviving life. My husband was making six figures we were living in a beautiful home. I volunteered and then worked in the recovery program for a large church. We had 150-200 participants every Friday night. We ate together, heard a teaching, and then split out into small, issue-specific groups. I loved both doing my individual work and working there. My boss had been my friend and mentor before I was brought on staff. On the surface, it looked like I was doing better than surviving.

The bottom completely fell out. All illusions were shattered. My husband fell into opioid addiction through treatment for chronic pain. As we were in the process of losing everything, our son presented with extreme, medicine-resistant, clinical depression. He was hospitalized multiple times for suicide attempts, suicidal ideation, paranoia, and delusions. My carefully crafted and managed world was collapsing around me, and there was no managing it. I was in a full-on post-traumatic stress disorder (PTSD) episode. My memory was nonexistent; I was making ridiculous mistakes at work. It felt like no one understood the full extent of what was happening. I talked to my boss, telling her what was going on at the time. My son was in the hospital, again. My husband was spiraling out of control. We were losing our home. I was falling apart. Her response? I will never forget those words. "Don't let anyone or anything steal your joy." It was crushing. It felt like she was telling me that I wasn't allowed to have the feelings I was having, and if I did, well then, my faith was not strong enough. Shortly after that, I was fired from the church, to both my great horror and relief.

How the hell was I supposed to find joy in the middle of all this chaos and heartbreak? I attended another church in town. I had been listening to the pastor online for a few months and thought it might be a good fit. I didn't expect much. Our family had been completely abandoned by our church home. I felt betrayed, and I was angry. It felt like my whole being was on fire. However, there was a flyer at the new church for a silent contemplative prayer retreat the next weekend. They had me at silent.

It was the beginning of my journey into the holistic healing world. The retreat consisted of group silent prayer, teachings, and individual quiet time. I walked the labyrinth several times. I listened to teachings about connection with people and all of God's creation. I sat in group prayer and watched as others struggled with being silent and listening. We did it together. On the last day and last group of the retreat, I knew. I knew that this was how to find joy during all of the chaos. No one was telling me how I should be feeling and maybe they still didn't understand the extent of what was happening, but they sat with me. The fire was beginning to cool.

I had practiced yoga for years as a physical exercise. I returned to it to get back to a manageable life. I know, I'm kinda stubborn like that. I wanted my life back. I still didn't understand fully that this shift was permanent. What I had missed in my previous yoga practice was spirituality, philosophy, and meditation—the whole healing that was available to me. While learning the westernized mental health system for my son, I was going deeper into my individual healing through yoga and contemplative prayer. What I was learning was that there was no one way to healing. This was piecemeal work. I had to find the right healing modality for me. I began learning about energy work, the chakras, and how we can apply it to ourselves and others. This was only the beginning of a beautiful journey of healing for my family and me.

I have nothing but the deepest gratitude for the therapists, psychiatrists, and medical doctors who treated our family through the years. Every single one of them wanted to help and did everything they were capable of in trying to support us. They were a part of our healing journey, and I do not ever want to diminish their work. Many of them were open to us seeking alternative treatments.

My healing had to begin with slowing down. Everything felt like an emergency. Time felt out of control. I felt out of control. Pranayama (breathwork) and meditation were invaluable in helping to regulate my sympathetic nervous system. Yoga asanas (poses) helped to ground me physically. The combination created the space in me to slow down and begin to look at additional modalities. I realized how important this was for treating severe trauma responses. I pursued and received my yoga teaching certification. I wanted to share this with the domestic violence survivors that I worked with. I also wanted more. I wanted to learn more, heal more, teach more.

I was introduced to Reiki through a friend. What a breakthrough! I was blessed to be taught by the late Angel Salathe. She was kind, compassionate, empathetic, and a lover of all people. She taught me about the healing energy available to all of us. She taught me about the chakras and how we carry particular types of energy in different parts of our bodies. She taught me about the connection between disease in our bodies and the connection to this energy and our environments. She told me to keep seeking healing, that being healed is not a destination for us humans; it is a constant state that we live in. She encouraged me so seek out any and all modalities that would help not only me, but also my family. She introduced me to shamanic philosophy around mental health issues, which led me to look at plant medicines used therapeutically to treat PTSD and depression.

My husband and I researched different treatments and how they were being administered in our area. He found a clinic that was using Ketamine with somatic therapy to help treat depression. He had been in a five-year slump while battling, addiction, anxiety, and depression. He agreed to begin the treatment. I had been talking with a friend about my PTSD struggles and was invited to a shamanic ceremony using plant medicines. Neither of us knew what to expect. Both of our journeys were led and guided by trusted mental health professionals.

Our experiences and healing looked completely different. His was a slow process. His treatments were scattered over multiple weeks. Unfortunately, the treatments were expensive, and he had to discontinue them before his big breakthrough. However, I did notice a difference. He was laughing at small things—something he hadn't done in years. It would be months before the big breakthrough would come. I am convinced that the treatments that he received helped to thin the wall of guilt, shame, and grief that had overtaken him. Once the breakthrough came, his healing was thorough and fast. My treatments were less frequent. I attended several ceremonies over a two-year period. With excellent guidance, I was able to walk through the trauma that my body was holding. I was able to face the core parts of my story that were keeping me locked in place, in need of all that control. I was able to completely release the stone that had been sitting in my belly for as long as I could remember.

This healing was messy for both of us. There is no fast track. I tried multiple other modalities in my search for healing including: Acupuncture, Rolfing, hypnosis, Emotional Freedom Technique (EFT), Aroma Freedom Technique (AFT), aromatherapy, and different types of massage. All of which were beneficial in their individual ways. Regardless of the modality, we still had to face the experiences and pain that were causing the suffering that we were each living with. Things didn't turn out the way we thought they would, the way either of us would have expressed the desire for at the beginning of this journey. We are no longer married. We are still good friends supporting each other through each of our healing journeys.

What I have absolutely loved in this journey is meeting people who are all for healing no matter what the journey looks like for each individual. Each of my teachers and mentors has emphasized a whole person approach, incorporating energetic healing, talk therapy, spiritual guidance, exercise, diet, and the need to be connected to nature. I live in deep gratitude for each of my teachers. I live in gratitude that the teaching did not end with my healing. I was encouraged to learn the practices that most helped me and to pass on the healing. This is how we heal the world.

I have learned a deep respect for healers who practice a myriad of modalities. I understand now there is no one size fits all to healing of any kind. I use Reiki, indigenous healing practices, and deep storytelling in my practice. I am still learning and seeking knowledge that I might one day be able to pass on to others.

I am often asked about the contradictions between my faith and the practices that I have used for healing myself and others. There is no contradiction. My faith was in the wrong place. It was in the people of a religious organization. My faith has only deepened in learning about these ancient practices. I see Christ in every person that has taught me and that I have taught. I see the intrinsic beauty of people and nature and how it was all created to work together. In nature and in ourselves, we have everything we need to heal. There are no magic pills that are going to heal the pain of our world. I am not anti-medication. I have seen cases where medicine is necessary and incredibly helpful. In all cases, we must find connection with each other and with the world that we live in. Holistic medicine is a beautiful gateway to the healing available when those connections are made.

Our son is doing extremely well. He has not yet tried the plant medicines. I don't know that he will. He's old enough to make that choice. What I do know is that watching us go through our healing processes helped him to stabilize and find individual healing. He has moved out and is living well. Never underestimate the power that your healing has on the people around you. I know that I will never question it again.

CHAPTER

Two

Help Your Body Heal Itself
By Angela Metropulos

ANGELA METROPULOS

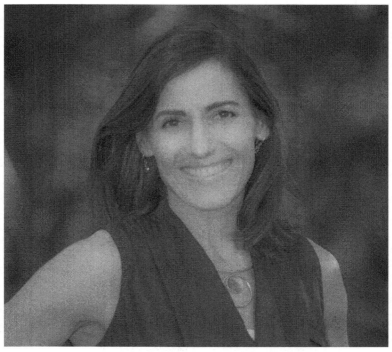

Angela Metropulos is a registered dietitian and integrative functional nutritionist specializing in mind-body healing, wellness and fitness, sports nutrition, and eating disorders. Angela's professional background includes serving as Director of Nutrition and Dietetics at several facilities, developing and teaching nutrition courses at the junior college level, serving as nutrition legislative coordinator, consulting, and holding private practices in Chicago, California, and Phoenix. Angela is also a professional speaker, registered yoga teacher, certified massage therapist, certified personal trainer, Reiki Master, and sound healer, and also teaches intuitive art classes. Connect with Angela on Facebook @Angela Metropulos or email angelametropulos@gmail.com.

Help Your Body Heal Itself
By Angela Metropulos

Holistic Healing: You Are a Holistic Healer

Your body has an amazing ability to heal itself. We have gotten used to going to doctors when we have aches and pains. What if we went within instead? What if we connected to the pain and asked our body what it was trying to tell us? What if we listened to what our bodies needed—the nourishment, cleansing, gentle movement, all the rest. What if we listened to the subtle hurts and intuitive hints?

No one knows your body better than you do. By ignoring the subtle symptoms, we allow the disease to continue until it is diagnosed. You are not your diagnosis. You have the ability to heal. Your body is actually a self-healing organism. It is equipped with natural self-repair mechanisms to fight infections, kill natural cancer cells produced every day, keep coronary arteries open, repair broken proteins, and defend against aging. *You* are actually your personal holistic healer.

What is Holistic Healing?

In general, conventional medicine focuses on treating physical symptoms; holistic medicine focuses on empowering people to heal themselves by improving the body's internal balance and flow of energy. Holistic healing is an integrative approach to health and wellness that focuses on the relationship between mind, body, and spirit, considering the entire person and the internal and external factors affecting them.

One of the biggest factors getting in the way of our body's natural healing ability is stress.

The Stress Response

Our autonomic nervous system has two major operating systems, the sympathetic nervous system, also known as *fight or flight*, which produces the body's stress response, and the parasympathetic nervous system, also known as *rest and digest*, which produces the body's relaxation response.

The stress response is the emergency reaction system of the body. This includes physical as well as thought responses to your perception of situations. Our stress response is there to save us—when our ancestors were chased by lions, the burst of adrenaline, epinephrine, and cortisol increased the heart rate and blood pressure and redirected blood flow to the extremities, activating large muscle groups to fight for their life or flee. Stress responses were meant to serve us in life-threatening situations; however, many of us are in fight-or-flight all the time. Our bodies are designed to handle small amounts of stress. It's the long-term, chronic stress that can cause extreme consequences.

The stress response can be activated when you are thinking about past or future events, and, it can be different for each individual. When we think about something stressful, the amygdala, a section of the brain which is responsible for emotional responses—especially fear—kicks into action and detects a threat, which initiates changes in our body such as increased muscle tension, rapid heartbeat, and faster breathing, which creates a vicious cycle where you become anxious and physically and emotionally over-whelmed. Every stressful thought disables the body's ability to repair itself. Feelings of loneliness can signal the amygdala to trigger stress responses as well as toxic relation-ships, childhood trauma, worry, and hunger, which sends the message that there is not enough food. The more stress you are under, the more your body functions in sympathetic or survival mode, which means that your body cannot heal. Your parasympathetic nervous system is where all healing takes place.

Below is a list of some common stress-related responses.

(Circle the symptoms you have had in the last week).

Physical

Headache

Dizziness/light-headed

Muscle aches/twitching

Stomach cramps

Constipation/diarrhea

Low energy

Increased heart rate

Chest tightness

Insomnia

Nausea

Chills/sweating

Hot flashes

Numbness in hands/feet

Dry throat

Neck pain

Increased urination

Weight gain/loss

Emotional

Anxiety

Anger

Agitation

Depression

Forgetfulness

Hopelessness

Guilt

Indecision

Insecurity

Increased sensitivity

Mood swings

Nightmares

Preoccupation

Racing thoughts

Worthlessness

Behavioral

Avoidance

Neglect

Teeth clenching

Poor appearance

Increased/decreased eating

Increased alcohol consumption

Fidgeting

Nail biting

Restlessness

Sexual problems

Withdrawal

Some people are better able to handle stress than others. If you circled several symptoms, you're likely in the stress response. It is a good time to look at how you're handling stress and add some positive coping mechanisms to enable the body's ability to repair itself.

The parasympathetic nervous system is designed to turn on your body's relaxation response. Getting your body and mind to relax for at least brief periods daily can help decrease stress responses and allow your body to heal.

My Story

Growing up, I always felt stressed. My mom was stressed, and we were always busy with a packed schedule of activities, rushing from one place to the other. I was super-sensitive. I could sense what others were feeling. I was sensitive to lights, sounds, noises, smells, feelings, crowds, everything. I had greater sensitivity to foods than others. All of this elicited the stress response in my body. That over-stimulation of the central nervous system caused my body to be in chronic stress mode.

I now know that I'm empathic. Being empathic means you can actually feel another person's emotions in your body. Since empaths are highly sensitive, their nerves can get frayed by loud noise, smells, or excessive talking and being around people can be draining. Many empaths are exhausted with adrenal fatigue since the adrenal glands are challenged by keeping up with the outside stressors, and the stress hormones get depleted. Symptoms include exhaustion, body aches, anxiety, trouble thinking clearly, and insomnia. Managing this sensitivity is crucial to keep the body in balance and out of fight-or-flight.

So what to do with all this sensitivity? I was guided to go to massage school when living in Napa, California, working as a clinical dietitian. This was the start of my holistic healing practice. I listened to my guidance over the years to learn Reiki and other energy healing modalities, study yoga, integrative nutrition, crystals, herbs, essential oils, and other alternative holistic healing methods.

The following are the top 21 techniques that I have used for myself and clients to keep the body and mind balanced:

1. Acupuncture

The practice of inserting thin needles into specific points throughout the body to restore the flow of qi, balance energy, promote relaxation, and stimulate healing.

2. Acupressure

The practice of applying manual pressure usually with the fingertips to manipulate the flow of qi energy to alleviate blockages that may contribute to health problems. Pressure points along the meridians throughout the body are linked with energy pathways attached to different organs and body parts, including the brain. You can stimulate acupressure points in your hands while sitting at your desk and in your feet by rolling them on a firm, small ball.

3. Art Therapy

Using a variety of art methods, including drawing, painting, sculpture, and collage, to express creatively and heal emotional trauma, violence, domestic abuse, anxiety, depression, and other psychological issues.

4. Ayurvedic Medicine

One of the world's oldest holistic/whole-body healing systems developed over 3,000 years ago in India, based on the belief that health depends on the balance between mind, body, and spirit, and that every person is made of five basic elements found in the universe: earth, fire, water, air, and space, which combine in the body to form three life forces, or *doshas*: Vata, Pitta, and Kapha, that control how your body works. The following are ayurvedic practices that can be incorporated into a healthy lifestyle:

- *Tongue scraping* stimulates internal organs through energetic connections with the rest of the body, improves digestion by increasing your sense of taste, and cleanses the body by removing toxins and bacteria from your oral cavity.

- *Dry skin brushing* stimulates the cells by increasing circulation, and breaks down toxins beneath the skin. It reduces stress, eases anxiety, and promotes relaxation.

- *Oil pulling* is the practice of swishing a tablespoon of oil, such as coconut or sesame, in the mouth for 10-20 minutes daily for oral detoxification. This may assist with bleeding gums, cracked lips, throat dryness, and tooth decay, in addition to strengthening gums and jaws, and whitening teeth. In ancient Ayurvedic texts, it claimed to cure headaches, migraines, asthma, and diabetes among other diseases.

- *Abyanga massage* is a full-body warm oil massage traditionally performed in the morning to dissolve accumulated stress and toxins in the mind and body, increase circulation, relieve fatigue, increase mental alertness, calm the joints, and nourish the body.

5. Balanced Diet

Nutrition can make a big difference in coping with stress and anxiety. Stress depletes your body of vitamins and minerals such as the B vitamins, Vitamin C, Vitamin E, calcium, and magnesium. These nutrients are released from the body to fight inflammation and neutralize free radicals created in response to stress and poor diet, which then weakens the immune system, making you more susceptible to illness and pathogens.

The following tips may help bring your body into balance.

- Eat a breakfast that includes protein. This helps to keep your blood sugar steady and improve your energy.

- Eat complex carbohydrates such as oatmeal and quinoa. This releases serotonin in your brain, which has a calming effect.

- Limit simple carbohydrates, such as sugary foods and drinks, which can spike blood sugar and anxiety levels and deplete vital micronutrients.

- Drink more water. This helps your body get rid of toxins and improves your mood and energy levels.

- Limit alcohol. This is considered a toxin in your system and can increase irritability and interfere with sleep.

- Limit or avoid caffeine. Caffeinated beverages can increase stress hormones and can interfere with sleep.

- Eat natural, whole foods and avoid processed foods. Eating fresh fruits, vegetables, and whole foods provides your body with the nutrients it needs as well as antioxidants, which help ease the symptoms of anxiety disorders. Spices with antioxidant and anti-anxiety properties include turmeric and ginger.

- Increase Omega-3 fatty acids. Primarily found in fish, eggs, walnuts, chia seeds, and flaxseeds, Omega-3 fatty acids inhibit the adrenal activation and cortisol elevation that occurs with mental stress.

- Supplement as needed. Since stress depletes vital nutrients needed to regulate the body processes, it may be helpful to supplement with a good quality multivitamin with minerals as well as omega-3 fatty acids.

6. Breath Therapy

Breathwork is a type of therapy that utilizes breathing exercises to improve mental, physical, and spiritual health. Somatic Breath-work Healing (SBH) utilizes a two-part pranayama breathing practice to bring the nervous system into an altered state of consciousness where stuck energies and emotions can be released.

7. Chiropractic

Chiropractic adjustments activate the parasympathetic system, which calms the fight-or-flight reaction triggered in the sympathetic system. The body's structure affects the rest of your body functions. Chiropractic adjustments release muscle tension, soothe irritated spinal nerves, and improve blood circulation, which can alert the brain to switch off the fight-or-flight response so the body can return to a relaxed state.

8. Crystals

Crystals can be used to calm the mind as well as absorb negative energy from your surroundings and from within yourself.

Best Healing Crystals for Stress and Anxiety

- *Amethyst* calms and relaxes the nerves and nourishes the nervous system, bringing clarity to the mind, relieving stress, soothing sadness, anger and anxiety, and balancing mood swings.

- *Sodalite* brings peace, calms the mind, and eases anxiety and panic attacks.

- *Kyanite* helps release anger, fear, and frustration, connects us with our higher wisdom, and aligns the body's chakras.

- *Howlite* resolves feelings of anger and helps with insomnia due to an overactive mind.

- *Moonstone* helps balance hormones, stabilizes emotions, and relieves stress.

- *Rose Quartz* promotes self-love and emotional harmony.

- *Shungite* acts as a shield from the electromagnetic fields emitted by computers, phones, and other electronic devices, which are a source of stress in the body.

- *Himalayan Salt Rock* eases tense, sore muscles and detoxes the body while removing negative energies. Use in a bath to ease stress, clear energy, and promote better sleep.

9. Essential Oils

Aromatherapy has been used since ancient times to promote feelings of calm and relaxation, reduce stress, insomnia, and depression by stimulating areas of the brain that are responsible for our emotions. Inhale, diffuse, or place on wrists or in a warm bath. Dilute 15 drops of essential oil for adults—three to six drops for children—with a carrier oil such as fractionated coconut oil, almond, or jojoba oil before applying to the skin.

Best Essential Oils for Stress and Anxiety

- *Basil* is treated as sacred in India for its highly beneficial properties. It reduces anxiety, fatigue, and depression and enhances clarity and peace by having a calming effect on the nervous system.

- *Bergamot* is used in traditional Chinese medicine to enhance the flow of energy, fight bacterial infections, and support digestive health. It is also known to enhance mood, promote joy, stimulate hormones, improve blood circulation, and balance the body.

- *Chamomile* reduces anxiety, regulates mood and stress levels, and calms the nervous system. It can also be used to reduce inflammation of the digestive tract.

- *Clary Sage* calms stress and anxiety, eases tension, balances hormones, reduces symptoms of PMS, and assists with depression by promoting inner peace. It also helps control cortisol levels, the stress hormone.

- *Frankincense* eases anxiety, improves depression, and helps to relieve pain.

- *Jasmine* promotes a sense of well-being and romance. Unlike some other essential oils used for anxiety, jasmine oil is thought to calm the nervous system without sleepiness.

- *Lavender* reduces anxiety, calms the nerves, and restores the nervous system. It also helps to lower blood pressure and heart rate and improve sleep.

- *Lemon Balm* has been used for hundreds of years for its medicinal and uplifting qualities. It calms the mind, reduces stress, anxiety, and depression, boosts immunity, and strengthens the nervous system.

- *Neroli* was used in ancient Egypt for healing the body and mind. It acts as a sedative, regulating the metabolic system and releasing feelings of anger, irritability, stress, anxiety, and worry.

- *Rose* soothes emotions during stress, grief, and depression, balances hormones and assists with headaches.

- *Valerian* enhances relaxation, calms nerves, and promotes sleep.

- *Vetiver* is used for anxiety and to promote relaxation, as well as having aphrodisiac qualities.

- *Ylang Ylang* lowers stress and anxiety levels, as well as heart rate and blood pressure and regulates cortisol levels.

10. Exercise

Exercise improves your mood by increasing the production of the brain's feel-good neurotransmitters, called endorphins, which reduces stress. It also lessens depression and anxiety and improves sleep. Only 30 minutes of exercise a day helps to reduce stress, anxiety, and depression.

11. Grounding

Nature is a powerful healer—walk barefoot on the ground, lay in the grass, touch a tree. Earthing (or grounding) transfers energy from the ground into the body for balance and healing.

12. Hypnosis

Hypnosis alters the state of consciousness and turns off the analytical left side of the brain, awakening the creativity of the right side. Hypnosis helps us overcome fears, withstand pain, and improve the ability to manage stress.

13. Massage Therapy

Massage loosens muscles, relieves tightness and stress, and increases blood flow throughout the body, helping to bring the body back into balance.

14. Meditation

Meditation helps with anxiety because it quiets an overactive brain. Even a few minutes a day of quieting the mind has profound results on your nervous system.

15. Music

Listening to quiet music has a relaxing effect on the mind and body, slowing the pulse and heart rate, lowering blood pressure, and decreasing the levels of stress hormones.

16. Naturopathy

Naturopathic medicine is a system of alternative medicine based on the theory that the body can be healed with nature, and diseases can be treated or prevented without prescription drugs, utilizing natural remedies such dietary and lifestyle changes, herbs and dietary supplements, exercise, acupuncture, and massage to heal the body.

17. Reiki

Reiki is a Japanese method for stress-reduction, relaxation, and healing that utilizes hands-on energy and the life force energy that flows inside of us.

18. Reflexology

Reflexology is applying pressure to certain reflex points on the feet, hands, or ears that connect to organs in our body. Reflexology is linked to treating headaches and migraines, cardiovascular problems, PMS, and sinusitis.

19. Sound Healing

Sound healing is the practice of using audio tones and vibrational frequencies to repair damaged tissues and cells within the body. It works on the idea that all matter is vibrating at specific frequencies, and sickness, disease, depression, and stress causes us to vibrate at a lower frequency. Sound healing utilizes singing bowls, gongs, tuning forks, and other healing instruments to promote relaxation. The sound vibrations impact our nervous system, engaging our relaxation, and inhibiting the stress response. The singing bowl tones synchronize with our brain waves, enhance awareness of the mind/body connection, and allow the body to shift into the parasympathetic nervous system, which slows the heart rate and calms the mind. Sound healing is beneficial for anxiety, depression, pain, PTSD, and stress as it assists with relaxation, clarity, balance, memory, and concentration, a stronger immune system, and improved sleep.

20. Sleep

Lack of sleep is one of the largest contributing factors to feeling stressed. Getting as much rest as you can on a regular basis is extremely healing and restorative. Turn off all technology the last couple hours before bed, pull the shades to keep the room dark or wear an eye mask for adequate melatonin production. Aim for eight to ten hours a night to promote healing.

21. Yoga

Yoga postures help ease the physical discomfort that is caused by anxiety as well as helping with anxious thoughts. A standing forward fold, *Uttanasana,* calms the mind while stretching and rejuvenating the whole body to reduce pain and stress.

These practices have helped keep me in balance so my body can do what it knows how to for healing. I encourage you to choose your favorite holistic healing practices and incorporate them into your daily life to reduce stress and activate your relaxation responses to turn on your body's natural self-repair mechanisms and help your body heal itself. You have the power to change your life.

CHAPTER

Three

A Mother's Awakening
By Becki Koon

BECKI KOON

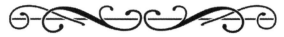

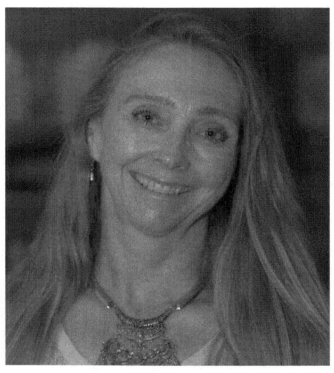

Becki Koon is a heart-based intuitive, transformational life coach, HeartMath Coach, Reiki Master, author, speaker, nonprofit consultant, and crystal practitioner. Through her business, Step Stone, Becki empowers people to activate, energize, and catalyze healing energies, reducing energy-depleting stress while assisting them in taking charge of their inner and outer worlds through remembering their divine essence. Becki's life-long search while raising a uniquely gifted, yet challenging and labeled child, led her to explore a variety of alternative healing practices. Many of those energy management tools/techniques made such a difference in her son's life (and hers and her family's), that she became a multi-faceted holistic healing practitioner with a passion for sharing energy awareness with those who are seeking a new way to experience their realities. You can reach Becki at stepstone2you@gmail.com or www.facebook.com/becki.koon.consulting or www.beckikoon.com.

Acknowledgments

I am honored to be the mother of two amazing souls, and I thank my son, T.J., and my daughter, Brandee, for choosing me to be their mom. My life forever changed by you entering my world, and the journey I now travel is a direct result of your teachings, wisdom, and love. Thank you, Jack, for sailing your ship in my direction so that we could navigate this part of our lives together, for lovingly pushing me to grow beyond my limitations and paradigms. To my parents Lionel and Kathy, I could not even imagine life without your love, support, and teaching me to be open-hearted to people, in service to others for a greater good. And a special thanks to my amazing mentors who opened doors showing me how to step into myself, my work, my reason for being: Lee Harris, Cheryl McCallister, and Lorie Ladd.

A Mother's Awakening
By Becki Koon

"**M**om, watch out," my son yelled from the passenger seat as I was driving down a lonely stretch of highway. Instantly my body tensed, adrenaline kicking in gear, and I was ready to hit the brakes. "Don't hit that lady," he frantically pleaded as I looked in the direction of his distress. He was pointing to the passenger side of the road. The air outside held a heavy mist, as the rain had fallen and then cleared a few minutes earlier, the road still wet with moisture. His worried eyes were searching my body to see if I was responding to the imminent danger ahead. For a moment, time stood still—and then he knew—that I did not see the lady alongside the road, who he had so clearly seen. There was a moment of eerie silence as we drove past the spot along the road that was empty of a visible woman. Skin-prickling chills started in the small of my back and ran up my neck. I wondered if she had seen him and knew he had seen her. I calmly asked him, "Did she see you?" I drove on as we sat in silence for a few moments. Once again, there was a strange awkwardness filling the air with this experience we had witnessed together.

By this time, when these occurrences took place, I gained composure and stayed calm, yet inquisitive to my son's sightings. They were as real to him as my physicality, and often, he could not distinguish one reality from another. I could only imagine what life was like for my twelve-year-old son, who had been through numerous emotional challenges already, to be a multi-dimensional seer at such a young and tender age. Seeing something you believe to be real and then recognizing that others do not see what you witnessed is not an easy thing to cope with at any age. A lot of people might say he was imagining these things; he wasn't seeing what he thought he saw, he was pretending. But I understood him like no other person in his life, and with a conviction I would later come to understand, I knew better.

"Yes, she saw me," he answered tentatively. "Is she still with you?" I asked. The moment I spoke those words, I had the feeling I already knew what the answer was. "She is still here with me." I was right, and my feelings confirmed. We were now delving into the realm of the unknown, for both of us were new travelers upon this untrodden path. I did the best I could to conceal my motherly concern as we jumped into a conversation that broke the uneasy silence.

These encounters were not always pleasing to my son. Sometimes they were downright frightening—for both of us. I was bracing and preparing myself to assist him without judgment with whatever unseen event was to unfold. I felt a bit like the blind leading the seer.

He began to squirm and wiggle in his seat, and suddenly, a huge smile erupted on his face. I breathed a big sigh of relief, as I knew that, at least this time, he was not frightened and this encounter was not disturbing to him. I decided to press him further gently. "If she is still here with you, then maybe you can ask her why? Does she have a message for you; something she wants to share with you?"

I had experienced this phenomenon with my son enough times to realize unwanted energy or attachments could occur, instantly and without invitation, and my deepest concern was for my son's well-being.

"She is here to fill me with unconditional love and to tell me that it is going to be okay. Her name is Linda, and she was a nurse. She was in a car accident when she was going home late one night. She was tired." He paused, and then quietly asked me, "You truly didn't see her, did you, Mom?" I glanced over at his big, blue eyes staring at me and slowly shook my head. The foggy mist seemed to add to the level of strange mystery and intrigue I was experiencing as I drove.

Then his whole body shifted, and he started to glow with brightness, happiness, and a smile as big as his whole face, while his body shivered and shook. I asked him what was happening and, beaming, he simply replied, "She just filled my whole body with love."

That was it. That was the end. She was gone, much to my mixed feelings of relief and awe. The conversation stopped, and we drove on down the road in still silence, my son contemplating what he had experienced, and I contemplating what I had witnessed.

It was an intriguing state of being for me, to be in a place of love, concern, and at times, fear for my child, while at the same time in awe, curiosity, and amazement about the paranormal experiences he was sharing with me.

Life with my son during those years was anything but mundane. And it wasn't only my son who was in life's picture, but my beautiful daughter as well, who reaped the reward, often unwanted, of an older brother who caught the attention of most people with whom he came in contact. The majority of that attention included an unease—the uneasiness of people who did not understand, were not aware, felt uncomfortable, and who judged first. The type of unease that arose when you couldn't put your finger on it, but you felt that this child was looking into your soul.

I knew from the time he was born that he was unique. The fact is we are all unique, but he was just more in your face about it. You couldn't ignore that unique aspect of who he was because he didn't give you the chance to ignore it. As a result, I became extremely adept at expecting the unexpected and not judging situations based solely on my limited perspective. Did I always succeed? Of course not, and at times, I would become completely exasperated by this unique child that seemed to take delight in pushing the envelope of accepted behaviors, beliefs, structures, and paradigms.

What I started to realize was that the unease of seeing my son go through the experience of not knowing one reality from another, ran way deeper within me than what was related to the current situation or event. There was a stirring down at the depths of my soul, a recognition, personal awareness of the state he was in. I had a sense and a deep knowing that I was experiencing much more than what my eyes could see.

I brushed it off as a mother's connection to her child. Isn't that how all mothers felt? Don't they all have that amazing empathy for their children; that heartfelt connection that aches when they see their children go through trials and tribulations? Of course, most mothers do.

Yet, somehow I seemed so connected to the utter confusion that at times enveloped my son; I felt like my nerves were raw and exposed. When I started to ask myself why I was being so affected, my mind and body responded by switching into automatic pilot. The plane of my uneasy reality was taking off, landing gear up, and I was flying away from the uncomfortable vulnerability I was not ready to recognize and feel. My focus would then shift to curiosity about my son's experience, insulated from my internal rumblings.

For many years now, I have shared with others my extraordinary awakening due to the amazing and sometimes tumultuous life I lived with my unique child—a child who challenged, and often still challenges, the heart of my belief systems, and the framework on which I had built my reality. The blessing is that the challenges I faced awakened me to the amazing and wondrous journey into holistic health and wellness that I now experience as a heart-based intuitive. I recognized who I was along the way, and it feels wonderful to be able to say it out loud, "Yes, I am an empath, heart-centered intuitive." It feeds my soul to be in a profession of passionately helping other people who are seeking a different or alternative way to view and understand their lives.

There are numerous energetic tools/techniques I learned to use in support of my son's sensitivities that have translated into my practice when working with clients. Many of those techniques I became certified to share, many others were a natural part of my gifts of healing. I will discuss a couple of the most useful energy management tools/techniques I found work for my clients and me, and then follow-up with an activity you can do for yourself.

Begin to recognize that everything is energy, frequency, and light. Awareness is a huge energetic tool that sheds light on thoughts, beliefs, patterns, paradigms, and issues so they can be seen and moved through us or transformed. Our third-dimensional, dense bodies feel solid, and we interface with a world around us that has perceived structure. That is real. But what is also real is that we are energetic beings, and that we are wired for remembering the multi-dimensional aspect of ourselves while here on this planet. That multidimensional aspect includes our physical body, mental body, emotional body, and etheric/spiritual body.

I had no choice but to begin to recognize the multi-dimensional aspects of life for my son and me to survive his reality; I had to open up my awareness to see in terms of energy flow and dimensional realities. I began to visualize energy around people and things using a soft eye focus, which helped me expand into understanding that all humans can learn to work with the various energy fields. When I saw the amazing, waving electric-blue field of energy above a mountain range, I was in awe. When I saw the waves of energy flowing around someone's body, I knew I was in alignment with my internal calling. I also learned to work with my higher self and guide network, calling on energies for the highest good.

Begin to look at everything in your world as energy in motion. You will recognize how we impact each other, how your actions go out into the field of awareness for others to experience, how others affect you even when no words are exchanged. Think about the smile of a stranger while you are waiting in line at the grocery store. It lifts the energy at that moment, doesn't it? It touches your soul at a deep, heartfelt level. This is energy flow in its simplest form.

Another energetic tool is the acknowledgment of your divine nature, connection to source. One of the biggest honors we can give ourselves is the gift of loving acceptance toward our divine uniqueness, knowing we are here on track and on purpose no matter how hard it may seem at times. The exterior circumstances surrounding our lives are not who we are. Call it whatever name that resonates in your reality, but the fact is this, if you are breathing air, you have divinity within you. We are heroic to be on the planet during this time in these dense bodies, while learning to navigate as divine energetic beings who can tap into other realities, other fields of consciousness.

We live in unprecedented times. Our lives are busier, faster, and more stressed than at any other time in history; yet we are at an amazing crossroads in our evolutionary process that is ripe with glorious potential. We can learn to breathe into who we are meant to be. By becoming conscious of our breath, we can learn to work with our body's mechanisms for stress reduction. We reset our physiological response and move into a state of balance. That state of balance brings us closer to our divine nature.

Here is an activity we can do anywhere, anytime, and in any situation. As we travel on this journey into deeper and often magical aspects of ourselves, we would do well to remember that our third-dimensional bodies could use our attention, especially in lieu of the fact that we live a reality in which we experience relationships, family, children, jobs, careers, responsibilities, health, wellness, awakening, sensitivities—the list goes on and on. What better way to be present for ourselves, than to perform conscious breath amidst it all?

Activity

- Become conscious of your breath, feel your breath.

- Breathe in and out a little slower and deeper than usual at whatever rhythm is comfortable for you. Perhaps five seconds in and five seconds out.

- Imagine that your breath is flowing in and out of your heart or chest area.

- Let your heart breathe in, breathe in the life force energy that is all around you and breathe out your stress, concern, worry, fear.

- If it feels right at the moment, you can exhale a little longer, releasing whatever needs to move out of your body and energetic field.

Do this breathing with or without your eyes closed, in the moment of life happening. Focus for one minute or several. Follow the dictate of the situation, it matters not. Just do it! It resets your autonomic nervous system response, moving from a chaotic physiological state into a balanced state. I know; it seems too easy. Trust me when I say, you do not need to make this complicated. Conscious breathing is a powerful tool in helping you navigate your world through all the ups and downs that come your way.

My breath became part of my toolkit while assisting my son through moments of uncertainty. The more balanced I became in my body, the more at ease he felt in his. It was as if that calming was contagious.

Be kind to yourself. Remember who you are—you are a powerful energetic being experiencing a heroic journey of self-discovery. You are never alone despite the planes of desolation you might feel. There are those of us who are working to support you in a holistic and balanced way. Seek us out. We are all connected, a part of the soup that makes up this journey, and when we can express our unique flavor in the world, that soup becomes a delicacy.

The plane of my reality has a welcome excitement, and this pilot's unease has lifted. I find the wisdom gained through allowing my vulnerability to be felt and acknow-ledged, is a gift I have the privilege to share with others. This journey, this path, this flight, is taking off and, ready or not, we are all in this plane of existence together. You are not alone!

CHAPTER

Four

Heal Yourself From Within
By Carla Hannon

CARLA HANNON

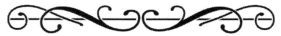

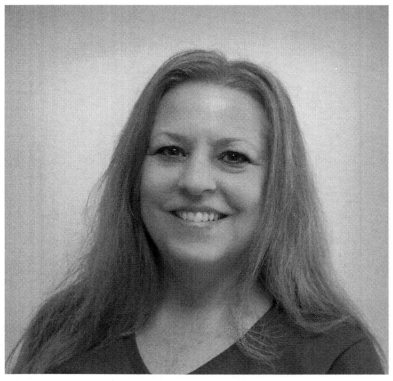

Carla Hannon is a 500 RYT with nearly 2,000 teaching hours, Ayurveda Health Counselor (650 training hours), Thai Yoga Bodyworker, and Reiki Master. Carla is a lifetime yogi, discovering yoga while running track and cross country. Carla practiced yoga throughout most of her life, which led to her pursuit for her yoga teacher training. She sought her Ayurveda Health Counselor training after discovering the unending benefits from both of these ancient practices in her body. Carla owns a studio, Balance Me Yoga, located in York, Pennsylvania, where she teaches yoga, meets with clients for private yoga sessions, Ayurveda Counseling, and Thai Yoga bodywork, as well as Reiki sessions, where she helps people live in their best life possible. She loves to learn and will forever be a student. Contact Carla by telephone 717-424-8948, or email balancemeyoga@aol.com. Please visit her webpage for more information: balancemeyoga.com.

Acknowledgments

I would like to thank Tony Marano for his unending support and encouragement in helping me to pursue my yoga teacher training and Ayurveda Health Counseling certificates. He has always encouraged me, even when I doubted myself the most. I would also like to thank my dearest friends who have stood by me and put up with my unavailability as I've studied so hard these last few years. I wish to thank my wonderful sweet yoga community—your encouragement, support, questions, and curiosity are why I continue to pursue more knowledge so I can share this ancient natural practice of self-healing. I thank each and every one of you from the bottom of my heart and send so much love and gratitude to you. I want to thank Kyra and Todd Schaefer of As You Wish Publishing for the opportunity for my first leap into writing.

Heal Yourself From Within
By Carla Hannon

I'll tell you a little bit about myself, and how yoga and Ayurveda have changed my life. I was a distance runner throughout high school and after graduation. At that time, my coach would give strengthening and stretching exercises to help keep me limber. After I graduated, I still did the exercises. My running had taken a back seat to life for the most part, but I always felt better with the exercises. I eventually figured out some of it was yoga—what the heck was yoga? Well, I started digging deeper, and found VHS tapes—yes, I'm that old. I would practice with my tapes every day, and I started developing a personal yoga practice, eventually without the tapes. At that time, there were only a few yoga studios, and I would go when time and money permitted. The wonderful thing about yoga is, I could do yoga wherever I was. I didn't need special equipment, a mat, maybe, but not necessary.

For the most part, I kept my practice throughout my life. I started learning about meditation, and I felt better physically and mentally. I've struggled with depression, anxiety, and other issues over the years. As life progressed, my yoga practiced evolved. I went from the hard, fast, and hot yoga to the gentler, flowing movement of Vinyasa yoga and the stillness of Yin yoga, taking my practice further inward. I can't tell you enough about the benefits to my body, as well as my mind, with this slowing down. My depression became less, I felt better overall, I became calmer, and my anxiety was slowly getting better too. I was

46

doing other things, too, without knowing what they were. I was using this little pot, called a neti-pot, for allergies. I started tongue scraping and oiling my body. Where did that knowledge come from? I truly don't know; I simply did it and felt better. This led to an in-depth study of yoga and Ayurveda.

Questions for you:

1. Have you ever had problems sleeping, either with insomnia or sleeping what could be considered too much?
2. Does your mind race, do you have thoughts that never stop going around in your head?
3. Do you have body aches and pains?
4. Do you have tight muscles?
5. Does your stomach get upset, either with or without eating?
6. Do you ever have skin rashes?
7. Do you have too frequent or infrequent urination or bowel movements? Do you know what the "normal" should be for your body?
8. Do you suffer from a stuffy nose or seasonal allergies?
9. Did you know digging a little deeper into these answers and talking with an Ayurveda Health Counselor can set you on the path to living in your best health?
10. What's stopping you from reaching your best health?

What if I told you I can help you with that? Would you take the time for yourself to learn about a science that could help you have good health, and hopefully avoid serious issues in the future? Yoga and Ayurveda can help you do that for yourself.

Yoga and Ayurveda are based on over 5,000-year-old systems, the *Yoga Sutras*, and *Charaka*. Yoga helps to achieve balance through movement, breathing, and meditation. Ayurveda brings daily practices, food, and herbs to help improve or maintain your good health.

Charaka Swastha

"One who is established in Self, who has balanced dosas (primary life force), balanced agni (fire of digestion), properly formed dhatus (tissues), proper elimination of malas (waste products), well-functioning bodily processes, and whose mind, soul, and senses are full of bliss, is called a healthy person."

Yes, yoga is the physical practice of the *asana*, or movement, and that is what brings most people onto their mat. The physical practice of yoga is great for the body by lengthening and strengthening muscles, finding balance, and overall physical well-being. But yoga goes beyond that—a regular practice of yoga encompasses not only the physical practice, but breath work, meditation, and body awareness.

The sister science of yoga is Ayurveda or *science of life*. The focus of Ayurveda is to live your best life without disease. Ayurveda focuses on disease prevention, versus the Western medicine focus on treatment, which is usually after a person has reached the disease state. Ayurveda consists of daily practices called *dinacharya*. This consists of daily care of mind, digestion, skin, teeth—basically, the entire body.

What can you expect when you meet with me, an Ayurveda Health Counselor/yoga teacher? The first thing I do with any client is a general intake. I'll ask why you are here to see me, and what I can help you with. I'll ask you questions about what time you wake and go to sleep, and what and when you eat every day. I'll observe your skin, and I'll look at your tongue. The real fun questions begin when we talk about your poop. Yes, I'll ask how often you poop, how you feel when you go, and what it looks like. But I will learn so much about you with these few questions. My intake is more involved, but these are the keys points, truly the starting point to putting you on your path to maintaining and/or improving your health. It's not crazy science or voodoo, it's guiding you to tune into your body and your mind truly.

My favorite part of working with a new client is helping them to figure out what they may need. Sometimes they come to me with a hunch that something is wrong or becoming out of balance, that somehow, they could feel better either physically or mentally. I love guiding them and helping them to choose their best options that fit their lives.

Let me tell you about a client I've been working with. When she first came to me, she was over-weight, barely sleeping, claimed to have regular bowel movements. She said she ate healthily, always ate vegetables, usually salads, and her one vice she would not give up was coffee, which got her through the day.

Fortunately, she came to me through her yoga practice, so this part was a little easier for me. Her assignment for yoga was to have a grounded practice. I encouraged her to come to my Yin class regularly and gave her a short home practice to do to satisfy her need for movement, but more importantly, a physical practice to help her feel grounded.

Upon talking and getting to know her even better, I finally got her to tell me about her true lack of bowel movements. Once or twice a week? Wow, she had to be uncomfortable. My goal from the beginning was to get her regulated once I learned how infrequently she had bowel movements. If I could accomplish that small thing, the rest would most likely fall into place. In the past, she tended to skip breakfast, and all she would eat was a salad for lunch and dinner, which had completely shut down her digestive system. So, we started simply, instead of her constantly eating salads and cold foods, I had her add a small breakfast, usually oatmeal or a small piece of toast with ghee or avocado to start her digestive process earlier in her day. I had her starting to roast her vegetables, which made them easier to digest, and we added ghee to her vegetables for lubrication to have the bowel movement. In addition to the roasted vegetables at lunch, I had her add some protein; she liked chicken, so she would roast chicken as well. I also had her add a *Churna* (a spice mix with the six tastes for her constitution) to her food to further aid in her digestion. Lunch needed to be her biggest meal, so she would have chicken and vegetables midday, sometimes with rice or quinoa for additional sustenance. For dinner, she would have soup, often with roasted vegetables added to a lighter broth-based soup. At the end of the day, lighter is better for digestion as your body is slowing down and getting ready for the night's rest.

With her coffee, I had her add some coconut oil, again, for lubrication, at first, she was reluctant, but now she enjoys the taste. I'm not a coffee drinker, but I understand this is pretty yummy. So, after a few weeks of only these few changes, I asked about her poop. She was now pooping daily, and her belly felt better.

After that success, we talked about her sleep, or lack of sleep, and how her mind constantly raced. This would be a tougher problem to help her overcome. So, we started simple. I had her sit in stillness each day, not necessarily meditating, but observing her mind and what was going through it at that time. I had her write down five things that came to her mind—not to address or "fix" them—just make note of them. That was a week-long exercise, then we talked again. I didn't tell her to do anything with the notes, just keep them and set them aside for later if she felt compelled to do something.

She also tended to be a night owl, staying up well past midnight and sleeping until 8:00 a.m., if her schedule allowed. This was a little difficult for her. Her tendency, if she couldn't immediately fall asleep, was to get up and do something—usually play on her cell phone. I told her no electronics, such as cell phone or computer, after 8:00 p.m. I asked her to go to bed every night, but 10:00 p.m. was lights out. I also asked her to get up and out of bed by 6:00 a.m. She wanted to sleep better, so she committed to it for me (actually for herself.) After two weeks, we touched base again, and guess what? She was rested and sleeping better, getting a lot accomplished every day because she was no longer so tired, and was starting to have routines. As her sleep and eating improved, her weight naturally started to regulate itself. She feels so much better and often tells me how happy she is to have found yoga and Ayurveda in her life.

So, here are a few quick tips to start today:

1. Sleep regularly. Wake and get out of bed by 6:00 a.m., and get to bed with lights out by 10:00 p.m.
2. For the most part, eat warm foods, eating your biggest meal at lunchtime, and adding six tastes with Churna.
3. Sit in stillness every day. Observe how you feel physically and mentally. Is it hard for you to be in stillness? Does your mind become a little quieter? Is it hard for your mind to become quieter? Take notes on how this feels for you.

Ayurveda isn't a miracle science, it's a self-practice—a self-study on how you operate both physically and mentally. Ayurveda is not one size fits all, it's what works for you. The beauty of yoga and Ayurveda is that we figure out how you operate and incorporate practices for you. We help you discover your constitution or *Dosha*, as we call it in Sanskrit. By asking my questions at your initial intake, I get a better idea of how to help you. There are three Doshas in Ayurveda, *Vata* (movement), *Pitta* (transformation), and *Kapha* (building). Everyone has one predominant Dosha, a secondary sub-Dosha, and a little bit of the third Dosha. Doshas are governed by the five elements—air, ether, fire, water, and earth. We need all five to live; therefore, we have all three

Doshas within us. Food, water, and tastes are also made of elements. Once I figure out your predominant Dosha, I can then figure out the best way to help you. For example, my client was Vata predominant. They are the movers; they get things done. Vata is responsible for getting us physically from one place to another, but also the internal function of our bodies, the breath, the elimination of waste, and the moving of blood within us. My client barely had bowel movements; however, once I helped heal her digestion by roasting her vegetables, adding Churna, and making the food quicker to digest, her bowels started to move better. Once I slowed her body and mind down by having her sit in stillness and not doing something all of the time, her mind settled down. By giving her a regular sleep and eating routine, her body and mind began to crave the rest and learned to slow down.

Ayurveda also focuses on how and when we eat. I mentioned trying to eat your biggest meal mid-day. By doing so, you give your body all day long—your most awake period of time—to digest and assimilate the food for your body. Ayurveda also suggests bringing all six tastes into every meal. The tastes are sweet, sour, salty, pungent, astringent, and bitter. It sounds strange, I know, but it's completely achievable in the form of Churnas made specifically for each Dosha. By using spices and incorporating all six tastes to your meals, you will wake up your taste buds, improve digestion, and better assimilate and use the nutrients from your food within your body, achieving overall good health.

Ayurveda also includes natural herbs, not only for use in foods, such as the Churnas, but to assist if needed for significant issues. For example, most people have black pepper in their pantry, but did you know it is fantastic for our digestion, circulation, and respiration? For digestion, it creates heat in our digestive fire to help our body digest quicker and move the nutrients into our circulatory system, improving our blood. For respiration, it helps to heat and dry things out, especially for those with upper respiratory issues. Do you notice how, if you have too much pepper, your nose runs? It loosens up the mucus and allows it to leave your body!

After learning about and incorporating holistic care for myself, I have never felt better physically, for the most part. We all get aches and pains, colds, or whatever, but overall, I feel better. I wish I had understood this sooner; I could have avoided years of using an asthma inhaler and allergy medicines, since I now have my allergies abated by using a neti-pot, I rarely have asthma attacks. I no longer suffer from seasonal allergies. By having a regular nighttime sleep routine, my sleep is better, I'm rested and accomplish more throughout the day, as I feel focused. It's when I don't follow my dinacharya I notice I don't feel as good.

Make the decision now to take control of your health, in whatever way is best for you. Do your research, interview practitioners that resonate with you. Make that best choice for you, whatever it may be. Live in your best health poss-ible.

CHAPTER

Five

Dying Well: It's Not An Oxymoron
By Cindy Kaufman

CINDY KAUFMAN

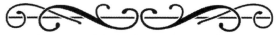

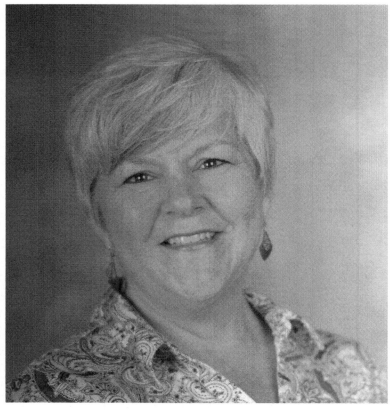

Cindy Kaufman, MEd, EdS, brings her background in counselor education, as well as her more than 20 years as a hospice volunteer, to her work as a Certified End of Life Doula, death educator, and writer. Cindy is the owner of HeartSpeak End of Life Companioning LLC. She serves as a compassionate companion on life's final journey for those with a terminal illness, assisting with life review, legacy work, and vigil planning, as well as providing caregiver support and respite. Cindy is also an ordained interfaith minister, officiating ceremonies, funerals, memorials, and life celebrations of all kinds. She is trained in home funerals and green burials, and she can guide clients who want these options. Cindy is based in Denver, Colorado, and can be reached at 720-989-1929, cindy@heartspeak2u.com, or www.heartspeak2u.com.

Acknowledgments

I extend my heartfelt appreciation to Michael, my husband, whose encouragement, advice, and love serves to propel me forward, not only as an author but with just about everything else I accomplish as well. To my daughters, Stacey and Lindsey, thank you for making my life so beautiful and meaningful. To Kyra Schaefer, my publisher, and Todd Schaefer, my editor, I extend my deepest gratitude for building the path so that I could find my way to realizing my life-long dream of being a published author. Finally, to my grandmother, Jeanne, with whom I sat my first vigil and experienced my first death, thank you. I miss you every day, Gram, but you are the reason I can do the work I do to help the people I help.

Dying Well: It's Not An Oxymoron
By Cindy Kaufman

"If I'm going to die, the best way to prepare is to quiet my mind and open my heart. If I'm going to live, the best way to prepare for it is to quiet my mind and open my heart."
Ram Dass

What is more holistic than living and dying, the totality of our existence? They are inextricably linked, for everything that lives will die, and everything that dies has lived, for however brief or for however long. Many authors write about living well, but few write about dying well. Why? Because we mortals, particularly in Western society, have a hard time with death. We avoid talking about it, thinking about it, planning for it and, most of all, seeing it. I'm guessing that right about now you are considering turning to the next section in this book and avoiding this article altogether, yes? I get it, but I ask you to bear with me. My goal is to help ease the discomfort of the topic and to help you approach the subject of dying well as easily as you approach the subject of living well.

"Dying well" is not an oxymoron. "Well" is not being used as a synonym for healthy, but as a synonym for satisfactorily. I promise, this article won't be morose be-cause I don't see death that way, and I hope that after reading this, you won't either. I acknowledge that it can take courage to contemplate our reality of mortality, but my dear brave reader, I encourage you to read on.

I work in the field of death and dying as an End of Life Doula (EOLD), work that I describe as "being a compassionate companion on life's final journey." It gets awkward when, in casual conversation, someone asks, "What do you do?" I respond, "I companion the dying." The reaction? Wide eyes, taken aback and often followed by an "Oh wow" expression. I smile without saying a word, and continue to let it sink in. Often the person will then say something like, "I don't know how you can do that. That must be hard work." The truth is that I do this work because it isn't hard for me. I'm drawn to it, and no, I'm not weird! It may seem cliché, but it is my "life's calling."

This work is truly rewarding for me. I am permitted to enter the sacred space at the end of another person's life and companion him or her, as I have been privileged to do many times over in more than 20 years as a hospice volunteer and now more recently as an EOLD. I approach each client as though I am the student, and he is my teacher. I may be familiar with death and dying, but I am not the expert on his life. I have much to be taught. If he is breathing, he is a living person. Thus, I focus on him living well while also dying well, for he is living while simultaneously dying. Indeed, aren't we all?

Life and death are inexplicably linked for the entirety of our lives, but we live as though they are not…unless we are faced with a serious illness, receive a terminal diagnosis, or are aging into our later years. In those times, we become aware of our mortal holistic duality of living and dying, but they are already synchronous throughout our lives. No matter how much we ignore the fact that we are going to die, it will happen at some point with 100% certainty, whether we have days or decades to live. Why not acknowledge this reality of our mortality, get comfortable with our ultimate destiny, and plan for dying well? I am not suggesting that we should remain focused on our eventual death every day (that would be morose), but accepting the reality of our mortality keeps us grounded in the present moment and at peace with what will, one day, certainly come. One of my favorite reminders is, "Talking about sex won't make you pregnant, just as talking about death won't make you die." So, are you still with me? Good! Let's look at one way EOLDs help others plan for dying well.

I would like to share the story of my work with "Mary." When I met Mary, she was residing in a skilled nursing facility where she had been for approximately two months. She had become terminally ill and could no longer live independently. Mary had been told that she had a couple of months to live, but because of family circumstances, no one could take her in and care for her in their home. Within those two months, Mary became bedbound because of her disease and resulting weakness. She spent her days lying in bed, staring out of the window, watching the birds fly back and forth to a feeder. It was her only form of entertainment. She had a television, but she was not interested in watching it. She wasn't much of a reader, and her eyesight was failing, so she didn't care to have books and declined to have someone read to her. She could either stare out the window at the birds, stare at the wall in front of her, or at the ceiling above her. Her waking hours were spent impatiently waiting for someone to visit her, especially her daughter, who would come by faithfully at the end of her workday.

Mary was anxious because that two-month deadline, as she called it, had passed and she was still alive. She did not want to be there, and she could not understand why she had not died. She was not peaceful with her circumstance. For a short time, she questioned whether her diagnosis was correct, but she had been placed on hospice service and was assured her prognosis was accurate. She ruminated incessantly on the fact that two months had gone by and she was still alive. She was approaching her third month of waiting, day after day, to die. She was ready, and she was despondent.

Mary's son enlisted my services as an EOLD, and I began to visit with Mary two or three times a week. I listened as she shared her story in whatever way it arrived, teaching me about her life, and building rapport and trust between us. I companioned Mary on her final journey for several months, a journey that turned out to be a lot longer than she had first anticipated. I learned what movies she liked, and I brought them in for us to watch together. I learned what music she enjoyed, and I brought some in for us to listen to together. I taught Mary how to use guided meditation to take herself to other places when she felt particularly anxious, places of her choosing where she felt love and joy and peace, places that held happy memories, even though she never physically left her room. This was something she could do for herself when she was alone, something that gave her a feeling of empowerment in a situation that was completely disempowering. She could not physically leave the room, but she could mentally take herself anywhere in the world and time-travel back in her memories.

Additionally, Mary's faith was of comfort to her, and we talked about her beliefs and what would happen when she died, where she would go, what it would look like, and who would be there. Mary envisioned that she would arrive in heaven and be welcomed by her husband, who had died 20 years before. The anticipation of being with her beloved husband once again made her smile and tremble at the thought of it. I encouraged her to go there in her mind's eye when she felt lonely. Over the next month or so, Mary's mood began to improve, by my observation, by her own report, and by the feedback I received from her adult children. Her anxiety was subsiding, and she was excited for me to know how the guided meditations were helping her. She expressed this to her children as well, and they communicated to me that Mary looked forward to our visits, as did I.

In addition to helping Mary gain a sense of empowerment over her living situation, I also wanted her to have empowerment over her dying situation. I introduced the idea of doing a legacy project, something we could work on together, that would be left for her children and grandchildren to remember her by. We brainstormed ideas, even something as simple as leaving letters for her family members that I could transcribe for her. She decided she didn't want to do any kind of legacy project. I acknowledged her decision, letting her know that the ultimate empowerment is the ability to say no to something you don't want to do. Next, I described doing a vigil plan whereby she could say how she wanted her final days and hours of life to be. She could not change where she would die, but she could decide who she wanted to be there, how she wanted her room to be, and any special instructions she would like for ritual at the time of her death. This was an idea that appealed to her, and she asked her children to meet with us so they could be present when she laid forth her vigil plan.

I scheduled a meeting with all of us, and we sat with Mary while she designed her vigil plan. I drafted the plan she wanted and placed it in her room for everyone to see. This experience was so rewarding for her children that they did not hesitate to begin setting forth her wishes the next day. They brought in her special quilt that she wanted on her bed. They brought her favorite bedside lamp and family photos to hang on the wall. They brought an oil diffuser so she could smell her favorite lilac scent. They brought family photo albums and old home movies, and I watched with tears in my eyes as they reviewed them with her while she was still alive to enjoy them. They laughed and marveled over memories they had long since forgotten. This activity brought them all closer together. Mary got to hear her husband's voice on the home movies, and the children got to hear their father's voice, for the first time in 20 years! They brought Mary's life to her room, and they brought life back to Mary. Mary's room was transformed into her home. It looked familiar, felt familiar, and the quality of Mary's life improved that day.

In the last few weeks of Mary's life, she felt less alone and despondent. I began to visit more often as her health declined further, as did her family. One day as I was leaving, Mary took my hand and said, "You are my angel, my earth angel. I want you to be with me when I die. I want you to walk with me into heaven. I want you to place my hand in my husband's hand as he reaches for me. Will you do that? Will you be with me?" I responded, "Mary, it would be my great honor! I will do everything I can to be with you when you die. I can't promise, but I will try my best to be here." About ten days later, I received a call in the middle of the night. Mary was transitioning, and I raced to be by her side, arriving as she took her final breaths. In my mind's eye, I handed Mary's hand to her husband as he reached out for her hand in heaven. Those of us present in the room held hands, recited the 23rd Psalm, and played the song, "Amazing Grace." This was the ritual Mary had designed for her vigil at the time of her death. My work of companioning Mary was complete.

Brave reader, I suggest you take a moment here and close your eyes. Take a deep breath in and let it out forcefully, as if releasing a big sigh. Relax with your eyes closed and focus on your breathing as you let go of any emotions around Mary and her story. You are in this current moment, and there is nothing sad here in this space. When you are ready, open your eyes and read on.

Below is an activity for you to do on your own. You can do this activity at any point in your life to begin making your plan for dying well, and in doing so, also contribute to your living well. Inextricably linked, remember? You don't have to be facing a serious illness, diagnosed with a terminal disease or aging into your later years to do this. This activity can be done by any adult at any age. If you are young and healthy, you can repeat this exercise again as you age, have experiences, and grow. Your answers may change over time, thereby revising your dying well plan for living well.

A DYING WELL PLAN FOR LIVING WELL

Name:_____**Date:**_____

What core values do you find most admirable in others and in yourself? (circle all that apply, add your own)

Authenticity
Achievement
Adventure
Autonomy
Balance
Bravery
Citizenship
Compassion
Community
Creativity
Curiosity
Determination
Fairness
Faith
Freedom
Friendship
Fun
Growth
Happiness
Honesty
Humor
Integrity
Justice
Joyfulness
Kindness
Knowledge

Leadership
Learning
Love
Loyalty
Optimism
Philanthropy
Reputation
Respect
Responsibility
Self-Respect
Service
Spirituality
Stability
Success
Wealth
Wisdom
Other: _____   _____   _____

How do you want to be remembered after you die?

(contemplate and write your response as thoroughly as you can)

I want to be remembered as someone who:

_____
_____
_____

Review your responses above and ask yourself the following questions:

Am I living in alignment with my core values and how I want to be remembered after I die? (contemplate and write your response)

_____

_____

_____

What steps do I need to take to become more in alignment with my set of core values (living well) and with how I want to be remembered (dying well), if I am not already? (contemplate and write your response below)

Step 1:_____

Step 2: _____

Step 3: _____

Step 4: _____

By signing below, I am making a contract with myself to take the necessary steps for living well and dying well.

Signature:_____**Date:** _____

CHAPTER

Six

Clarity, Truth And Self-Liberation: How To Live A Unique Life And Still Fit In
By Donna Kiel

DONNA KIEL

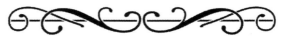

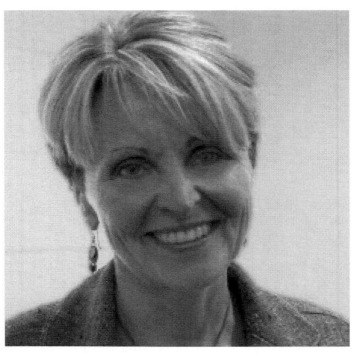

Donna Kiel has dedicated her life to helping others achieve their highest and truest potential, and find passion and purpose in life. As a counselor, teacher, principal, life coach, and mentor, Donna has inspired thousands in gaining self-awareness and achieving greater levels of personal and professional success. She holds three degrees, including a BA in psychology, an MA in counseling, and a doctorate in leadership. Donna's approach provides a practical method of self-assessment that can be applied every day to confidently live a life of meaningful purpose. Donna's specialties include compassionate leadership, innovative organizational change, team building, personal transformation, loss and crisis resolution, and mediation. Donna works with individuals and groups through her services as a mentor, coach, workshop leader, and consultant. Donna offers free assessment and consultation for those seeking growth. She can be reached at drdonnakiel@gmail.com or through her website at www.donnakiel.com.

Acknowledgments

In all our lives, there are times when we stumble, fall, and lose our way. It is the compassion of others that lifts our soul and brings new light. My deepest gratitude to those in my life who have forgiven my imperfection, who have seen in me that which I could not, and who have given me the inspiration that became my words on the page. To my family, friends, colleagues, clients, and students, I thank you for sharing your hearts with me. To my greatest muse, my granddaughter, Charlotte Sue, your life gave my life new meaning and purpose, and with one smile, I found fearless love and the courage to speak my truth. I owe the deepest gratitude to my imperfection, fear, sorrow, and loss. Within each moment of suffering, I have found the greatest of teachers and the truth of mercy.

Clarity, Truth, and Self-Liberation: How to Live a Unique Life and Still Fit In
By Donna Kiel

"It is better to live your own destiny imperfectly than to live an imitation of somebody else's life with perfection."
— Anonymous, The Bhagavad Gita

Hidden behind our fear, self-doubt, need to belong, and our longing to have a perfect life are pearls of inner wisdom and truth.

Life is a series of choices. We make choices based on our conception of what is right. Sometimes our choices come at the cost of denying our dreams, because we believe we are choosing what we *should* choose and doing what we *should* do. Our lives can become busy, productive representations of an image of the right life. We may end up choosing the important-sounding job, the culturally acceptable relationship, and the house that looks good, all the while feeling a longing for more.

On a personal note, I have always felt like a misfit in a world where everyone else seemed to fall seamlessly into a category of a cultural group. For a long time, I struggled to understand who I am, where I fit in, and what I was meant to do. The only thing I knew for sure is I wanted my life to help others, and I wanted to belong.

My need to belong led me to try on all sorts of cultural costumes and play many roles throughout my life. I adopted the role of counselor, teacher, mother, and school principal. I found that I could be whatever anyone needed me to be. You see, I *needed* to feel accepted, liked, important, and needed—and I did. I also longed for something more.

We humans often make life a complicated struggle. When our heart says one thing, and our mind says something else, it ignites a battle of epic proportions. For as long as I can remember, this battle has been raging inside of me. I have always wanted to fit in, and yet I also had a deep longing for something else.

When our culturally conditioned minds are connected to our mouths, our hearts don't stand a chance in being heard. I often have said yes when I meant no, only to feel like I fit in, was important, or had a life of value. Fitting in and saying yes to others made me feel the connection I longed to experience.

Often, we are told we cannot have it all in life. Many theories say to follow your heart—you must let go of the mind's need for cultural acceptance. I could never do that. I coached hundreds of clients who cannot do it either. I have a high need to fit in, and I have a high need to listen to my heart. Along the path to do both, I have discovered it is possible to fit in and follow your dreams. The clarity, truth, and self-liberation required to follow your heart can also guide you to fitting into the next place where you belong. The key is listening to your heart's call.

Sometimes, if we are lucky, and when we least expect it, the heart's call sets in motion cataclysmic events. That hard-won moment is something to cherish and act on.

For me, the moment occurred in the most unexpected circumstance as I was ending my first year as the principal in a new public school. I was experiencing great success. I had a great faculty, wonderful parents, and students who were succeeding. There was no logical reason for me to be paralyzed by the question, "What do you want?" Yet I was. I had nowhere to hide, and it felt as if every breath made me sink deeper in quicksand. I experienced the combo platter of confusion, rage, and shame, not to mention a side-dish of fear. What I wanted didn't matter.

My role as a principal was constantly busy. I didn't have time to want anything. My to-do list was pages long, including working on my doctorate, mom worries, and adjunct teaching at night. My life involved award-winning schmoozing, suit-wearing, constant organizing, and all the "stuff" that made me feel I fit in. It also consisted of shoving aside any suffering inside my heart.

After all, I was getting a great salary, I was making a difference in the lives of young people, I had a big title, and all the ego-boosting accolades I needed. Why would I ever see a disconnection between my mind and my heart's desires and dreams?

During this moment, my voice shook as I responded, "I don't know what I want." The emotion took over my body, or perhaps my body was finally taking over to get through to my mind. I began to weep and fell to my knees in the most primal pain. My body had said, "Enough of this." And then a faint voice whispered, "Stop, let go."

What was happening to me? Why was I unraveling when my life seemed perfect? Years later, my therapist asked me what I would say to the principal I was back then. In a voice of calm strength, I said, "Don't do it." It took me almost a decade to realize my breaking point had nothing to do with the job and everything to do with silencing my inner voice—my truest self.

I now know that moments of anguish are invitations to bravely and boldly find new meaning in your experience. To suffer is to want something to be different. All the while, our human conditioning has trained us to do everything we can to avoid suffering. It tells you to keep yourself busy with to-do lists, with saying yes when you want to say no, and doing all the *shoulds*. We are masters at how to avoid suffering.

In truth, suffering that takes the form of fear, longing, sorrow, or anger can be wonderful and transformative. Suffering is our best opportunity for self-liberation and realizing our dreams. Getting your mind to align with your heart often requires suffering. We all suffer. Whether suffering is mourning the loss of a loved one, or worrying about a snarky email, we suffer. We enter suffering in the nanosecond that it takes our mind to create a story of doom. Yet, each moment of suffering can unlock the dreams that create the next best version of you.

In my life, and in my teaching and coaching of hundreds of people, I have discovered a simple, practical formula to help us to use our suffering for transformation.

Three Steps to Self-Liberation

While working as a newbie high school counselor and teacher, I stumbled upon taking complex ideas and breaking them down into three main points. After lots of failures and long-winded, confusing lectures (where even I felt like I was about to fall asleep), I realized everything I taught could be broken down into three main points. It worked every time. Science supports the idea that we remember small bits of information better than long, complex ideas.

What follows are three steps to gain clarity, truth, and to liberate yourself by getting your head and heart on the same page. I created the acronym AIM, which stands for acceptance, integrity, and mercy, as a way to remember the process, which consists of three steps to handle any moment when suffering mounts its attack.

Acceptance—Stay here now

Step one is to accept suffering and stop resistance or distraction. We distract ourselves from our suffering with work, complaining, over-analyzing, self-doubting, self-deprecating, and a million other ways. The first step to self-liberation is allowing the suffering to be present without blame or answers.

Whenever I feel my body tense up and heat surrounding my neck, I instinctively want to resist whatever painful thought has entered my mind. I want to distract, avoid, and run away from the suffering. These three simple words bring me back: "Stay here now."

As doing exercises stretches our muscles to make them stronger and comes with pain, suffering is the mandatory tax we pay to gain self-liberation. Our instinct is to flee or fight the suffering; however, *staying* in the suffering is vital to becoming your true self. Suffering is our heart's way of expressing that we are lying to ourselves, and it is our heart and our true self asking us to stop.

Integrity—Let's talk

Step two involves finding integrity and requires an honest, candid talk between our heart and our mind. That's right, we need the two parts of our inner world to talk to each other. While this may be an unconventional concept, it is grounded in spirituality and science. There is the mind that makes up beliefs, and the heart that is our unconscious truth.

Our mind can create all types of fear, resistance, and doubt. Our heart, however, is the speaker of truth. Having a discussion that lets your heart and mind have an equal forum to speak will surface the truth of what is going on. To have this discussion, I find it best to create an image or character of the *me* that is my heart and the *me* that is my head.

In more detail, I imagine my heart as a gorgeous woman, with a beautiful smile and big blue, compassionate eyes. She only wears comfortable, flowing clothes and never wears shoes. She is free. My mind, on the other hand, is dressed in a snappy business suit with a matching scarf, has perfectly styled hair, shoes with heels, a clipboard and lots of rules. She has a serious look and oversees all the details and degrees we have obtained.

To make the conversation between my mind and my heart as expedient and effective as possible, I created an acronym of the typical reasons why my mind may choose to ignore the desires of my heart. The acronym, ALIVE, gives you the key focus of topics that surface when the mind is trying to take over the heart. You can ask your mind and heart if what you are doing is to feel accepted, liked, important, valued, or engaged with others. The acronym

ALIVE represents each of the emotional needs that cause us to do things we may not want to do. ALIVE includes:

- Accepted
- Liked
- Important
- Valued
- Engaged

We each have imperfect lives. No matter where we came from or the wonderful parents we had or didn't have, we are all wounded. We spend our lives trying to find and then fill the emotional needs left by situations and circumstances that were never in our control. What I have discovered is that those early life wounds never go away. In fact, none of our wounds ever go away. Contrary to what you may think, this is not a bad thing. The needs we have are opportunities to become our best, most compassionate, and merciful versions of ourselves. Paradoxically, those emotional needs you avoid are the gifts that you bring to your best self.

For example, if you have a strong emotional need to be accepted and important (like I do), you may tend to work hard to please others. In the process, you are successful and do great things. You are fitting in, and that is not a bad thing. The key to aligning your head and heart is to understand that what you are doing is filling an emotional need, then you can make a choice that allows your heart to speak with integrity.

Circumstances can temporarily cloud our truth, but a candid discussion with our head and our heart can bring clarity. We are our best ally.

Mercy—I got you

Step three is to give yourself mercy. Mercy is this wonderful assurance that no matter what has happened, you are safe, forgiven, and loved. The best tool I have in my arsenal to sit with suffering is to reassure my (scared) self that I have my back. One of the most pivotal moments of my life happened when, as a principal, I was waist-deep in conflict with the school's faculty members. I believed my job was to make all the teachers and students happy. I'm pretty sure that was flawed thinking. Not surprisingly, this mindset left me emotionally and physically demolished after a faculty meeting, where faculty blamed me for their fears and failures. It was the mercy of one of the school's administrators that brought me back. As I sat in my office contemplating becoming a Walmart greeter, he stood in my doorway, looked at me, and said, "Hey, it's okay; I got you." His act of mercy brought me such a strong feeling of relief that I let out a flood of tears. I felt that I belonged and that someone could help me. That moment of true mercy transformed my entire being.

Within you is the person who has successfully navigated previous sufferings and all the hard stuff of life. Step three is giving yourself true mercy. It is vital to your everyday life to forgive and welcome home your *imperfectly perfect* mind and heart with gentle, loving, and compassionate mercy. Whenever I am confronted with turmoil, suffering, and the busy confusion of distraction, I pause and say, "Hey, I got you. It will be alright. I have been there and had your back through awful, terrible times, and I have your back now." Being merciful to ourselves is perhaps the most significant and meaningful key to liberating your true self.

Self-Liberation

This wonderful life of yours has an expiration date. Wasting time by avoiding pain or creating a hurried pace may not be the best use of your precious life. For me, self-liberation and finding clarity and truth are an ongoing process, but one that is well worth the hero's journey to get there.

I encourage you to accept suffering, find integrity by questioning whether what you are doing is keeping you ALIVE, and, finally, give yourself mercy. Be the person who says—unconditionally —"I've got you," and be the person who gives the gift of mercy to all other sufferers walking among us. Your time is now, there is no one on this planet like you, and your heart is calling you to liberate yourself, to gain clarity, and to awaken to its truths.

CHAPTER

Seven

Underlying Causes Of Ill Health
By Gwen Foster

GWEN FOSTER

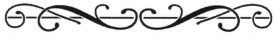

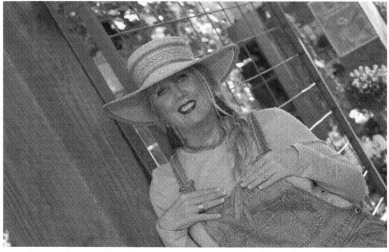

Gwen Foster is the owner of NuVision USA, a company that offers an advanced software program for natural health practitioners. Gwen created the data for NuVision and uses NuVision with all clients to help identify blocks and imbalances. Her passion is working on underlying emotional conflicts and triggers. Gwen also uses herbs, homeopathy, flower essences, essential oils, and nutrition to help her clients. Gwen is a Hanna Kroeger Practitioner, Certified Master Neuro-Linguistic Programming (NLP) Practitioner, hypnotherapist, and personal coach. She is also a Doctor of Naturopathy (ND) and Doctor of Natural Medicine (DNM). Gwen currently sees clients in Katy, Texas, and holds long-distance appointments as well. She loves to teach live classes on many health subjects and has free educational videos available on her YouTube channel. To contact Gwen, please call 281-236-5453 or email gwen@gfia.net. Find out more about NuVision at www.nuvisionusa.com.

Acknowledgments

I want to acknowledge Hanna Kroeger, my angel and inspiration. Her teachings have been a great source of information to help heal myself and others! I don't know what I would have done without her knowledge, and I don't know how effective I would have been with helping others without taking the Hanna classes almost 20 years ago. I also want to acknowledge my friends, family, and clients. I've learned more from them and their health journeys than any class or course! I appreciate their willingness to share their experiences and make changes in their lives. They are the real healers as they healed themselves!

Underlying Causes Of Ill Health
By Gwen Foster

I was lucky to find Hanna Kroeger's work 20 years ago when I was suffering from several chronic health issues including adult-onset asthma, recurring bronchitis and pneumonia, shingles, lupus, acid reflux, chronic fatigue, and fibromyalgia. I was on nine medications a day, and spent a lot of time at doctor appointments and in bed. In the 80s and 90s, I was on high doses of Prednisone for long periods. Back then, chronic fatigue and fibromyalgia were considered psychosomatic (in your head) and Prednisone was handed out like candy! Anyone suffering chronic fatigue or fibromyalgia know they are not crazy, and there can be some level of depression and/or anxiety about the way you feel the longer the symptoms persist.

Hanna Kroeger's teachings were hugely important in my full health recovery, and are an essential part of how I work with health clients today. Both allopathic doctors and some holistic health practitioners can focus on symptom management, which is like putting a Band-Aid on the wound. This does not resolve the underlying cause or reason the person has health challenges.

Hanna Kroeger's *7 Physical Causes of Ill Health*

Neglect (poor nutrition, dehydration, lack of exercise, lack of sunlight)

Congestion (of organs and glands)

Environmental toxins (including chemical and metal toxins in foods, pesticides, dental work, and in our environment)

Parasites (all types)

Infection (such as candida, parasites, bacteria)

Miasms (hereditary energetic residue of tuberculosis, syphilis, gonorrhea, and others)

Trauma (physical and mental)

And she believed that *emotional and spiritual trauma* also affect our physical health.

A few simple examples of neglect that can have a big impact on health symptoms, are mineral and amino acid deficiencies. A lot of people dealing with heart-related symptoms, such as arrhythmia, heart palpitations, and chest pain, are usually mineral deficient—especially of calcium, magnesium, potassium, and iron. Heart medications don't resolve the mineral deficiency, but are used to "manage" the symptoms. Restless leg, poor sleep, nervous system disorders, weight gain, anxiety, muscle spasms, and poor circulation may be caused by mineral deficiencies. Minerals are found in foods grown in the ground, and that's why a diet high in vegetables is important. Most Americans don't eat enough vegetables. Iceberg lettuce and a small portion of broccoli a few times a week won't cut it. One recent book, *Brain Body Diet*, says you should eat 11 servings (five to ten cups) of vegetables per day. Also, minerals don't absorb if a person is acidic, and most Americans are acidic. I perform lab interpretation for clients, and the most common lab factor that needs attention is acidosis, metabolic acidosis, or diabetic acidosis. These are all caused by a diet that is more acidic than alkaline. It's pretty easy to figure out—only fruits and vegetables are alkaline, and everything else is acidic. If you have toast or bagel or coffee or eggs for breakfast, these are all acidic. A sandwich or a salad with chicken and ranch dressing is also acidic. The steak or chicken and potato and wine are all acidic too. One or two servings of veggies per day cannot offset the rest of the acidic foods. And there is no way to offset a typical Mexican or Italian dinner.

There is a great quote in the book, *Modern Nutritional Diseases* by Ottoboni, that says, "A disease is not a disease if it can be healed with diet and nutrition!" Ottoboni is referring to type two diabetes, heart disease, stroke, obesity, and cancer.

Another great example is the kidneys. The kidneys control the pancreas (diabetes), which can be the underlying cause of hypertension, and can affect vision, the knees, and cause edema, water retention, and weight gain around the lower abdomen, hips, and thighs (saddlebags). Poor kidney function can also be the cause of low back pain.

If you are dealing with chronic illness, I would say the underlying cause has not been addressed or rectified. I've met numerous people that have been doing Lyme disease protocols for years. This tells me that Lyme is no longer the issue, and it's something else that has not been identified, or there is something else wrong that is not allowing the body to heal. In the case of chronic Lyme, it might be the person's constitution has not been addressed. If their body temperature (oral) is under 98.2, and they are acidic (pH under 6.8), they are a host that pathogens like and they will be hard to get rid of.

There is no magic pill that makes us well. Unfortunately, we have to make changes to our diet, and many times to our environment, to get well.

Emotional Causes

Another big influence in my health restoration was the realization and resolution of health problems that stemmed from past emotional conflicts. I had adult-onset asthma that required four medications. Three of them were daily inhalers, and I had one emergency inhaler. I could not exercise without having an asthma attack that made me feel like I was going to suffocate and depleted me energetically.

When I learned Neuro-Linguistic Programming (NLP), the instructor identified the adult-onset asthma was attributed to a bad breakup with a boyfriend who had cheated on me. I would have never believed it, but I was asthma-free within eight minutes and never used an inhaler again! Asthma can come from hyperventilating type crying. I have found this to be true in numerous cases of asthma due to a divorce or death of a loved one or pet. And the timeline made sense. I started having asthma attacks in the 90s, within a year of the breakup.

It was hard to grasp how I had taken medications for asthma for over ten years to find out it could be resolved in less than ten minutes, and the underlying cause was an unexpected and traumatic event with an ex-boyfriend.

I was aware of Louise Hay's work back then, but saying the affirmations and doing mirror work had not helped my actual health symptoms. At about the same time, I was learning NLP and hypnosis, I was made aware of Dr. Hamer's German New Medicine (GNM). The original GNM chart had mapped out the underlying emotional cause of most cancers. With some pretty simple questioning, I found it to be 100% accurately related to people I knew who had cancer.

Dr. Hamer's basic theory is that a *significant emotional event* (SEE) starts a series of biological responses in the body of all mammals, which are survival and protective mechanisms. Most humans don't realize or understand their health issues are messages from the body or biological responses to help them survive. We are honestly not a lot different than the dog that marks his territory by peeing all over the yard (incontinence) or concedes to the alpha of the herd (low hormones). It takes a while to understand German New Medicine, but it honestly explains most health dysfunction.

What is Your Body Trying to Tell You?

What if varicose veins were meant to make your legs stronger and help you stand up for yourself? What if incontinence was to help you mark your territory (home) from in-laws, stepchildren or overbearing parents? What if your low hormone production is to help you get along with the alpha personality at your job or home (co-worker or spouse)? What if your skin condition was to "toughen you up" to not be so "thin-skinned"? What if your digestive issues are related to that thing that is "eating at you"? What if your lack of sleep is giving you more time each day to resolve your issues?

What if your hearing is declining because of nagging, complaining, or negativity? What if your chronic fatigue is a "play dead" reflex because you can't cope with a certain situation, job, or marriage any longer? What if your memory is declining because of something that you did or something that happened to you in your past that you don't want to remember anymore? What if you have an issue that affects you having sex? What is your body telling you?

In my experience, people don't think of what their body is telling them, and most people will do almost anything not to make a change. Some people would rather suffer in an unsatisfying job or bad relationship than make a change. It's amazing how many people have experienced and endure emotional, physical, mental, and spiritual abuse, and stay in that situation versus being alone. I think the big elephant in the room is the denial of how these abusive relationships affect our health, but we are taught in modern society to take a pill for it. This subject could be an entirely separate book on how people, especially women, are conditioned to accept their circumstances even if it's to their health demise. We are taught through family patterns, religion, and social conditioning "to make it work" or "stick with it." And we also stay in these unhealthy situations due to low self-esteem, low confidence, and because of guilt or manipulation.

One childhood conflict can set up a person for numerous psychological and physical health complaints. If the original childhood event is not resolved, there is a cascade of additional physical and mental symptoms that can occur. When a child is sexually abused, it is common to have "constrictive" (or protective) mechanisms activate. This can include constipation, teeth clenching or grinding, TMJ, muscular contractions, and headaches (constrictive). A lot of times, there is also anxiety, depression, self-blame, guilt, and/or post-traumatic stress disorder (PTSD) symptoms. Related self-devaluation health conditions are common, such as fibromyalgia and arthritis, including rheumatoid arthritis. Other self-devaluation feelings can cause any bone or lymph conditions and varicose veins. And there can be any number of nervous system disorders, including anxiety. The nervous system is interesting because this is where I think the most Band-Aid approaches are used to alleviate symptoms without getting to the underlying cause. If someone has had a "fight or flight" or "survival" experience, the sympathetic nervous system activates. Imagine you are running for your life from a wild animal. There are certain biological responses that take over—your digestion is impaired because you not saying, "Hey tiger, let's stop so I can eat, chew my food thoroughly and digest my food," sleep is impaired because you are not saying "Hey tiger, stop chasing me so I can get a good night's sleep for eight hours and let's continue this tomorrow," and busy brain or ADD type symptoms occur because your brain is thinking quickly in a survival situation and is not focused on any long-term project.

After a while, the person is "wired and tired," where the nervous system is like the Energizer Bunny that keeps going and going, but the brain and physical body are exhausted. This sympathetic dominance can happen from a single traumatic event or a chronic stressful life. So, one traumatic event or a series of traumatic childhood or adult events can set up someone for many health problems.

And then there's the "straw that broke the camel's back," and that's when the bottom falls out. That's when the Energizer Bunny can't get out of bed. That's when the person can't take care of themselves or their family.

I give my clients homework if they are willing to examine the underlying emotional cause of their health problems. This is the exercise—write down all health problems and when they started. Try to use the date your symptoms started, but also include the diagnosis date (if you have one). Include hospital or emergency room visits. You might not remember the exact month and day, but make any date references you can, like junior high, senior year, or early 90's. Write down everything you can remember, even if the health symptoms are completely gone now. Leave a few lines of room between each health symptom and try to organize by date, with the most recent dates last. I like to do this in a Word document, so it's easy to edit and move things around.

Then, write down all traumatic events, especially unexpected events, like a car wreck, divorce, death of a loved one, death of a pet or friend, fired from a job, miscarriages, or abortions. Include dates you moved, especially if you didn't want to move. Also, include any dates of injuries (this could be your injury, your child's, or another person's), and burglaries or robberies. Then add other significant dates like when your children were born, when you got a new job, or when you remarried. Include events such as your parents' divorce (even if you were an adult), when you found out a loved one was diagnosed with cancer, and other bad news. Also, include significant relationship breakups and when new relationships started. Work on this for a few weeks on different days for the best results.

If you can't think of a significant event within 12 months before the beginning of a health issue, ask yourself what happened that year. The timeline you create can be extremely useful in gaining realizations about yourself and how your body has responded to emotional events. Your timeline can also help you heal by knowing what caused the symptoms, and help you navigate future responses to emotional events.

One last thing about Dr. Hamer's theories is that many times the health symptoms are after the resolution of a conflict, meaning when you meet the new man or woman to replace your ex or when you get the new job. When someone is in fight or flight, certain body functions are affected, which were described earlier. When there is a resolution, the body goes into parasympathetic dominance, which is when the pathogenic activity begins to clean up the mess from the "fight or flight" phase. Pathogens mean infections, including bacterial infections, urinary tract infections, yeast infections, and Lyme infections. Cancer diagnosis (fungus) and symptoms include chronic fatigue (recovery mode) in the recovery phase.

The body is *incredible* if we understand it and the messages it gives us related to our health symptoms. Wouldn't it be awesome if we could get a health symptom and immediately take action to resolve the conflict? And it would be helpful if we could forgive and forget those traumas and unexpected emotional events almost as soon as they happen so that we don't have to suffer! We've all heard that it's important to forgive because we are only hurting ourselves if we don't. I can tell you it is necessary to forgive, and you are only hurting yourself and your health by not forgiving. My opinion comes from 20-plus years of experience working on my health and with hundreds of people. I have also learned the importance of neutrality because of German New Medicine. The larger the amplitude of the crisis, the emotions, the ongoing talking about it, the lack of forgiveness, and the lack of letting go are the biggest factors of ongoing health problems!

CHAPTER

Eight

Saying Yes To Yoga
By Jan Wilson

JAN WILSON

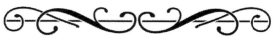

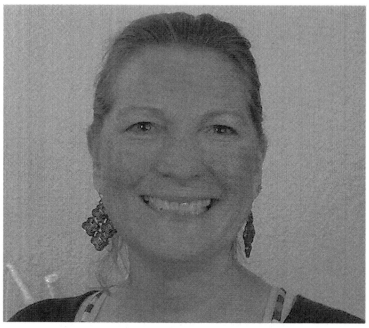

Jan Wilson is a 200-hour-trained yoga instructor, with additional specialized training in prenatal and aqua yoga. Jan also has additional training in acupressure, Reiki, and holistic nutrition. She was drawn to teaching yoga by the sense of connection, gratitude, and healing she felt in her practice. She assists individuals with increasing their mobility, and creating balance and stability within their body, mind, and spirit. Her passion is to demonstrate and teach that yoga is for every body. You can reach Jan at, every.body.matter@gmail.com, or through Facebook at https://www.facebook.com/EBMPE.

Acknowledgments

I would like to express my special thanks of gratitude to my teacher, Mary Simmons, as well as my fellow yogis, who gave me the support and opportunity to learn all that yoga has to offer, which helped me find the power within for finding peace, and the desire to help others do the same. With a special thank you to Maly Low, who continues to be an inspiration in my daily life.

Saying Yes To Yoga
By Jan Wilson

Embracing and succeeding with yoga is no different than with any change we desire. However, allowing change to fully incorporate itself within our lives cannot be accomplished overnight.

Prior to becoming a yoga instructor, I had severe spine and sciatic issues. The pain was often so strong that it would bring me to tears. During a visit with my chiropractor, he said, "Before we go to surgery, let's try physical therapy." I was afraid to be in pain for the rest of my life, yet there was no way that I wanted surgery. So, physical therapy it was.

From day one of my treatment, based on previous experience, I realized I was doing yoga. As my therapy progressed, I decided to return to a regular yoga practice, which I continued as my therapy ended. After six months of consistent yoga practice, there was no sign of pain, no fear of going on a hike in the mountains, and I was no longer concerned about aches after sitting for too long.

Now that I was pain-free, I realized that yoga was the key to my health and longevity. I began to study it in-depth, deepening my practice and bringing it fully into my life. Yoga poses date back over 5,000 years, and present-day yoga is based on the evolution of those teachers who came before us and passed down their teachings. Although most people associate yoga with the physical poses (also known as asanas), these poses or positions only make up one of the types of yogic practices. Any single or combination of types can create a happier, healthier life. These types are: meditation, karma, devotion, knowledge, mantra, and postures.

Meditation—Focus Grasshopper

A lot of people say they multitask, yet studies have shown that those simultaneously addressed tasks suffer and the end results never seem to be quite up to par. Meditation is taking time for a few moments to breathe. We all suffer some form of monkey brain—our minds are always jumping from one thought to another. Thankfully, meditation comes in a variety of forms—it can be silent, it can be a visual exercise, or can even be music or sound-based. The goal is to find what works for you.

All meditation asks you to do is focus. For instance, during silent meditation, you can focus on your breath, the flame of a candle, or whatever focal point helps you be in the now. Yes, your mind is going to try to take over; that's okay. When you realize that you're listening to the voices in your head, gently remind yourself of your focal point. Meditation takes practice, and your mind will wander until you become accustomed to your meditation. Remember, when your meditation period is done, it's done—no dwelling on how successful it was, no worrying about whether you did it right. It's over, let it go. Next time you may amaze yourself with the progress you've made. The healing power of meditation has even begun to find itself in schools, replacing detention.

Meditation can also lead to awareness, giving us the ability to be focused and always in the moment. Being aware is not an easy thing to maintain, and while a simple concept, can remain challenging. How often have you gone somewhere in your car and suddenly realized you don't remember any part of the drive? How often do you drive the same route to work and then notice something new, only to realize it's been there a long time? So often our awareness is not on the task at hand.

A daily activity to help you work on your awareness is the *yogi meal*. As with all things yogic, a yogi meal has its guidelines, which basically consists of common sense. Try it the next time you have a meal!

Always eat while seated. No talking with food in your mouth. While eating, unplug from external distraction. Focus on your meal, enjoy it, taste it. Completely finish chewing and swallowing before taking the next bite. Keep your servings to the size of two handfuls. If after finishing the first serving you feel unsatiated, wait a few minutes. If the hunger persists, add one handful and stop there. Wait at least two hours before your next meal. That's it. The way you eat, along with the portion of food eaten, will create a happier, healthier you. Of course, you should do your best to limit foods high in sugar and sodium, but all you need to do is to take your time, focus on your meal, and enjoy it.

Karma – Giving

When was the last time you treated yourself to a random act of kindness? Yes, it is a treat for you, not only the person receiving. How good does it feel when you give the perfect gift to someone? The joy on their face, their heartfelt thanks. Taking the opportunity to give back in the middle of your day can completely transform your outlook on life. It can provide continued movement toward a happier, healthier life.

I've found that opportunities for kindness are all around us, all the time. You don't have to look for them—be aware of life around you. When you give, you gain. And not from the receiver, but from others and from unexpected sources!

Devotion—Embrace Your Higher Power

Embrace your belief in a higher power, in whomever or whatever it is that guides you. Hold it close to your heart. I believe that practicing gratitude helps hold our devotion close. Whether you show your gratitude through deed or word, allow it to happen at least once a day conscientiously. You can say a short prayer in the morning, or in the evening, write down your words of thanks for the day you had.

Knowledge—Always A Student

To keep our minds and bodies fresh, we must be willing to learn from others and become a lifelong student. Take time to look up a word if you're unsure of the meaning. Ask questions when you don't know the answer. Be open to any opportunity for learning, whatever may present itself. If you don't have time when it happens, write it down and come back to it later. Take that online course or that cooking class. Try a new workout program. Find anything that appeals to you and learn, learn, learn!

Mantra—Listen to the Rhythm

Sound has tremendous healing properties and has been practiced by millions of people across cultures. You may already be practicing a mantra and not realize it. For anyone who has seen the movie or read the book, *The Help*, you may remember the scene where a small child is taught: "You is kind, you is sweet, you is important." That in itself is a beautiful, self-healing mantra. You can also use a mantra as your meditation.

When I was in a time of need, a dear friend shared a simple mantra with me; called Om Brzee Namaha. To practice, start by inhaling deeply. As you exhale, begin pronouncing, "Aum Breezy Naum A Ha." Without practice, it's unlikely you can finish it in one exhale, so breathe through it. Traditional yoga practitioners suggest repeating it 108 times, and there are ways to help you keep track. When starting out, I suggest that you repeat this as often as you feel necessary. You'll know when it's complete, and it's a great way to start your day. It's also another form of meditation.

Postures—Movement and Breath

When anyone mentions yoga, people think of taking the body into a variety of positions. Yoga can be done almost anywhere, not only in a studio or a heated room. People starting out can even practice in a swimming pool. It's important to understand that yoga should not cause pain. It may cause discomfort, but if it hurts, adjustments can be made to accommodate your body. Your asana yoga practice is what is right for you. It does not require the ability to put your feet behind your head—at least not in the beginning.

What some refer to as a yoga practice is a series of positions and movements connected to your breath. Yes, it's that simple! There are a variety of asana formats or practices, the key is to find the format that speaks to you, and to not let your brain rule your body, but then again, that could be said for everything we do.

In the years I've been teaching yoga, I've had practitioners from ages six to ninety, many of whom to this day continue to practice. In fact, I have taught classes where many of the practitioners can do positions with more ease than I, and of course, the opposite is true—I've taught practitioners who have chosen to do positions that I have no desire to do. Yoga, after all, is a personal practice. That is at the heart of understanding yoga. No two bodies are built the same—no one body is symmetrical. What can be done on one side will not necessarily be able to be done the same way on the other. I have two students who wanted to feel better and get stronger, and both stated that they were never able to touch their toes. After starting a regular practice, both could reach their toes at the end of five weeks.

The good news is you need not rely solely on your body when following a yoga asana practice. There are various pieces of equipment, referred to as props, to assist you. These props support our bodies, where necessary, until such time we no longer need them (if it's meant to be). We can use blankets, pillows, or foam blocks, to name a few. In fact, a full asana practice can be done while seated in a chair. The one piece of equipment I recommend to everyone is a yoga mat, also referred to as a sticky mat. It's "sticky" because it keeps you from slipping as you move from one position to another, and it can also be used to add cushioning between the body and the floor.

Yoga is so widespread that numerous formalized exercise programs include yoga positions. Many of us who have participated in other group fitness classes or obtained the services of a personal trainer have done yoga. Remember the stretches you did at the end of class or training? Their origin is yoga. In fact, as stated earlier, many physical therapy treatments include yoga positions to help with the body's healing process. Without even realizing it, yoga has already touched many of our lives.

As with life, breathing is a key part of the asana practice. Learning to connect with and become aware of our breath can provide improvement and healing to your body and your life. As with asanas, there are different methods with different benefits. Proper breathing should be learned from an experienced teacher.

I have a client who is a CPA. She does a lot of sitting, especially during tax season, and her tax season lasts well past the April 15th deadline. There were times when she experienced trouble standing and moving, once she stood from her chair. In fact, on more than one occasion, her husband had to wheel her around in her chair because she was in so much pain. She used the services of medical professionals, but it never seemed to help. After a month of regular asana practice, the pain reduced significantly. Now during her heavy tax season, she no longer fears sitting for hours upon hours. She knew that sticking to her practice would allow her body to not rebel against her.

A Daily Yoga Practice

Take sixty seconds to five minutes for a short meditation following the method that suits you. Focus on what's at hand, try a yogi meal once a day—enjoy and taste your food. Take the opportunity to enjoy a random act of kindness, either at the store or on the road, wherever the moment strikes. Learn something new—a word of the day, perhaps. Listen and embrace the sound around you, or listen to music and take time to focus on that sound. Do your best to remove any distractions. This could also be your mediation. Embrace

God or your higher power, and thank that power for what you have, either through prayer, a journal, one word, a full sentence, or a full page.

Find 15 to 60 minutes for an asana practice, one to two hours after a meal. If you are practicing first thing in the morning, do so before your first meal. Consider including one or more of the other yoga types into your asana practice.

Sun Salutation—An Asana Practice

Standing at the top of your mat, feet directly below your hip bones, arms relaxed by your sides, slightly bend the knees and gently tilt the tailbone forward. Take your awareness to your breath. Try to control your breath so that the inhale and exhale are the same length. A simple count of one, two, three for each can suffice. Each movement and each breath should work together. Allow your gaze to follow along with the movement.

1. Inhale and raise arms, palms facing each other. Gaze past the thumbs.
2. Exhale and fold forward from the waist, heart to your thighs. Gaze to the tip of your nose.
3. Inhale and rise halfway up, fingertips to knees or shins. Open the heart. Gaze past the third eye, the space between your eyebrows.
4. Exhale and plant the hands firmly outside the feet. Step or jump legs back to the top of a push-up. Lower your heart. Gaze at the tip of your nose.
5. Exhale and roll onto the tops of your feet, bringing shoulders back. Gaze past the third eye.
6. Exhale and tuck your toes under. Raise your hips and extend your back. Gaze at your navel or through the legs. Take five breaths. Relax and try to

move your weight to your legs. Try to find your best upside-down V. This is a supporting pose and your first downward-facing dog.

    a. You can also drop to your hands and knees first, and then lift the hips.

7. At the end of your fifth exhale, walk or jump your feet to your hands and raise the heart halfway, fingertips to knees or shins. Gaze past the third eye.

8. Exhale heart to thighs and fold forward. Gaze beyond the tip of your nose.

9. Inhale and raise your arms, palms facing each other. Gaze past the thumbs.

10. Exhale and release your arms to your sides or to heart center placing palms together and gaze to the tip of your nose.

The extent of healing that I and others have received through regular yoga practice goes beyond words. It is with a grateful heart that I offer thanks for each and every one of us!

CHAPTER

Nine

Laughter Yoga: A Slice Of Heaven
By Janet Carroll, RN

JANET CARROLL, RN

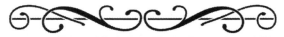

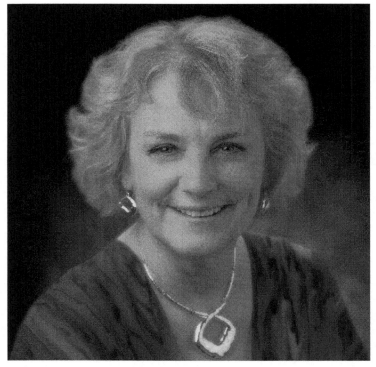

Janet Carroll has had an impressive triad career including 48 years in nursing, 35 years in massage therapy, and five and a half years in Laughter Yoga. This has given her not only decades of experience in health services, but also special insight into health and well-being on all levels: physically, mentally, and emotionally. It is from those experiences, and her passion for assisting others in healing their lives, that her transformational programs, classes, and presentations were birthed. Her focus is health, happiness, and healing through Laughter Yoga. Janet's accumulated skills allow her to engage her audiences in a way that combines both her wisdom and passion. She teaches fun and effective skills that can be shared, applied immediately, and continued throughout life. You can reach Janet at Janet@JanetCarrollRN.com. Thank You!

Acknowledgments

There are so many people who have graced my life and have helped me to become who I am today. To all of you, you have my deepest appreciation! The dearest of them all are: my son, Dominic Burch; my daughter, Stephanie Archuleta; my granddaughter, Javielynn Archuleta; my sisters, Barbara and Sheila; my brothers, Larry and Paul; my mother and father; Grandma and Grandpa Schmitt; my teacher, William David; my ND/Iridologist/Herbalist and consultant, Mickey Jones; my editor, Dawn Greenfield Ireland; and my friends, Linda Ballesteros, Mikole Montgomery, and Donna Owens. I am extremely grateful!

Laughter Yoga: A Slice Of Heaven
By Janet Carroll, RN

"Heaven is not a place after you die. It's a vibration you
can access while you are alive." ~Abraham Hicks

It all started with a short repetitive dream ten years ago.
There I was, in a large auditorium, addressing a full-to-
capacity audience. As I am leading the group, everyone
is laughing *hysterically*, nonstop, for the entire dream!
Almost as though Robin Williams was performing! In
reflection, I have a fun sense of humor, but the laughter in
my dream was way beyond my comedic abilities. I would
always awaken from my dream with question marks floating
through my mind. I had no clue as to how to interpret this
dream.

The dream repeated itself approximately once every
three to four months for five years. After those five years of
dreams, I discovered Laughter Yoga and—voila! I
immediately knew that Laughter Yoga was for me. I now
lead various groups in the healing art of Laughter Yoga.
And, yes, a lot of the groups I present do laugh
hysterically—exactly like in my dream!

I have never smiled or laughed as much as I laugh now
and I love it! I am so happy to share Laughter Yoga. It
appears to me that most of the people in the world are starved
for laughter. I feel so lucky to be a part of a world-wide
laughter community committed to bringing laughter to the
world with a goal of health, happiness, and world peace.

Question: What is joyous, fun, free-of-charge, can be practiced any time, any place, alone or with someone?

Answer: Laughter Yoga! Yay!

Here is information on the basics of Laughter Yoga:

"Laughter Yoga is a single exercise routine that reduces physical, mental, and emotional stress simultaneously." ~ Dr. Madan Kataria, MD, Founder of Laughter Yoga

1. Laughter Yoga is based on the concept that anyone can laugh for no reason, without jokes, humor, or comedy
2. We initiate laughter as an exercise in a group, but with eye contact and childlike playfulness, it soon turns into real and contagious laughter.
3. Laughter Yoga combines laughter exercises with deep yoga breathing. This brings additional oxygen to the body and brain so you can feel energetic and healthy.
4. Laughter Yoga is based on the scientific fact that the body cannot differentiate between fake or real laughter. You receive the same physiologic and psychologic benefits—fake or real!
5. Laughter Yoga was started in 1995 in Mumbai, India by Dr. Madan Kataria (a medical doctor), and has since grown to six of the seven continents.

Laughter Yoga is now practiced all over the world and is still rapidly growing. It is in companies, corporations, schools, colleges and universities, senior centers, hospitals, healthcare settings, and any place where people work or gather. It can also be practiced alone.

Here's what happens in a Laughter Yoga session:

1. Laughter exercises
2. Clapping
3. Deep breathing
4. Childlike playfulness
5. Laughing, singing, and dancing

Laughter Yoga is fun and easy! There are no skills to learn, and no special clothes, shoes, or equipment required. You are an expert from your first session!

Stress

Stress is a physical, mental, or emotional factor that causes bodily or mental tension. *Stresses* can be external (from the environment, psychological, or social situations) or internal (illness, or from a medical procedure). Shockingly, stress is a major factor in five of the six leading causes of death—heart disease, cancer, stroke, lung disease, and accidents. The body is wonderfully designed to handle our stress through the stress hormones of *adrenalin* and *cortisol*, and our adrenal glands handle it all. Located right above the kidneys, the adrenal glands release adrenalin during emergencies to give you superpower strength and courage to deal with dire emergencies.

During regular everyday stress, the adrenal glands:

- Release cortisol to help stabilize blood sugar levels
- Regulate metabolism
- Reduce inflammation
- Reduce blood pressure
- Assist in memory, and balance the sodium and water in our bodies

The problem is that we were never meant to be living in stress every day, all the time. Since most of us are under huge amounts of stress on a daily basis, our bodies try to help us out by releasing extra cortisol. Over time, the result can devastate the body with:

- High blood pressure
- High blood sugar
- Weight gain
- Loss of calcium from bones
- Depression
- Decreased immune function
- Loss of muscle mass
- Increased fat in the body
- Loss of memory and cognitive function

It throws your entire body out of balance! Overwhelming, isn't it?

Here's a fun metaphor for what we look like when we are in high levels of stress—the Peanuts character, Pig Pen, in Schulz's comics! If you remember, Pig Pen always walked around with a cloud of dirt swirling around his head and body. That's exactly what we look like when we are in the overwhelm of too much cortisol rushing through our bodies—we're enveloped in a big gray swirling cloud.

Good News: Laughter Yoga Can Help

But, before I venture into explaining how to apply Laughter Yoga in reducing cortisol, here's some basic information you need to know. There are two "roads" in life—the Red Road and the Blue Road.

The Red Road is labeled as the sympathetic nervous system prepares the body for intense physical activity and is often referred to as the *fight, flight, or freeze* response in the body. It's an emergency response system. The hormones of the Red Road are adrenalin and cortisol. The Red Road (adrenalin/elevated cortisol) can cause havoc on your body in the following ways:

- Accelerated heart rate
- Widened bronchial passages
- Decreased movement of the large intestine
- Constricted blood vessels
- Increased peristalsis in the esophagus
- Dilated pupils
- Causes goosebumps and sweating
- Elevated blood pressure

The Blue Road is labeled as the parasympathetic nervous system, which has the exact opposite effect of relaxing the body and inhibiting or slowing down many high energy functions. We refer to the main hormones of the Blue Road as the "happiness hormones," which are endorphins (happiness), serotonin (relaxation), dopamine (motivation and love) and oxytocin (bonding). The happiness hormones bring relaxation, satisfying and regenerative sleep, joy, peacefulness, being grounded and centered, meditative, creative, and much more!

Special note: Because women are hard-wired differently than men, and because women must deal with emotions and feelings, it is imperative that women ground and center in the Blue Road every day.

How to Move from the Red Road to the Blue Road

Now, I'd like you to reflect on your personal stress patterns. What symptoms do you go through as you accelerate from stress to distress?

My experience is that stress/cortisol will build into distress when the stress continues over a long period of time, culminating in an emotional explosion. For me, my big warning signs are irritability and overwhelm. I can handle stress, but sometimes it sneaks up on me. This is why I do 15 minutes of preventative Laughter Yoga every morning so that I can manage my stress.

I have learned to recognize my stress patterns, and when the irritability and overwhelm starts, I "get it," and immediately start the following routine to stop the excess cortisol flowing through my veins and get grounded, centered and happy again.

The Key is Your Sound and Your Breath

1. Take a deep breath in through your nose or mouth and make an *Ahhhhhhh* sound as you inhale. Slowly count to five.
2. Release that breath slowly through your mouth as you make an audible *Haaaaaaa* sound as you exhale. Slowly count to five.
3. Repeat three times.

Next, add a smile. Here's why—when you contract the muscles around your mouth, cheeks, and eyes in a smile, the seventh cranial nerve sends a message to the brain that you are smiling. Then, the hypothalamus tells the pituitary gland to release endorphins (natural opioids) into the bloodstream and you start feeling awesome!

1. Now, please put it all together:
2. Inhale deeply and slowly with an *Ahhhhhh* sound to the count of five.
3. Smile (fake or real). Continue your smile as you exhale slowly with a loud *Haaaaaaa* sound to the count of five.
4. Repeat three to ten times.

By this time, you should begin to feel better. You have started the process to stop the excess cortisol and open the door to the Blue Road of happiness hormones! Please remember that Laughter Yoga consists of deep breathing, laughter, singing, playfulness and/or dancing.

Now, it's time to perform Laughter Yoga exercises for 15 consecutive minutes or longer.

1. Laughter Yoga is flexible—you may sit or stand.
2. You may do the exercises alone or with two or more people in a group— either in person, via Skype, or over the phone. It's usually more fun with several people.
3. If in person, most groups meet for 45-60 minutes

Note: There is evidence to suggest that if you do 15 consecutive minutes (or more) of laughter, singing, dancing, playing every day for six to eight weeks, you can reset your entire immune system! This is powerful, considering that the immune system is the bottom-line system in the body. If your immune system is open and flowing, it will bring health to the entire body.

Here's a fun secret I learned from my massage practice about how you can tell if you, or someone else, has entered the Blue Road of the happiness hormones, meaning no excess cortisol—they are grounded, centered and in the flow of life. Their eyes glow like bright headlights, and, generally, there is a slight Mona Lisa smile on their face!

Here are some of my favorite Laughter Yoga exercises:

1. Very Good! Very Good! Yay!
   This is extremely popular and fun to do with all age groups!
   - Do this exercise in between other Laughter Exercises
   - Chant loudly and smile as you clap hands and say: "Very Good! Very Good!"
   - And, as you raise your arms above your head, say: "Yay!" Repeat as often as you like.
2. The Two-Year-Old Tantrum
   This is the most popular exercise that I lead. All age groups love it, and many women go out their way to tell me how clear, light, and happy they feel after their tantrum is over!
   - Stand or sit
   - Put both arms in the air, with fists clenched.
   - Anchor both feet on the floor/ground in a firm stance.
   - Count backward—three, two, one— then scream as loudly as you can, stomp your feet and flair your arms, exactly like a two-year-old!
   - Continue for ten seconds (or longer). Then, laugh for ten to fifteen seconds.

- Breathe deeply to re-ground and re-center. Doesn't that feel good?
3.   Song from Snow White and the Seven Dwarves
- It's time for a group sing-along!
- Hi Ho, Hi Ho, it's off to work we go
- Ho, ho, ho, ho, ho, ho, ho, ho
- Hi Ho, Hi Ho, Hi Ho
- Repeat four to five refrains as you smile and laugh!

4. Take a laughter pill and laugh non-stop for one full minute!

- You will be amazed at the sounds of the cycles of laughter you go through.
- Don't be afraid to add a little zip to your laughter and say a few "whoo hoos"

5. Cowboy Laughter: Yee-Haw! Knee Slap!

- Sit forward, or stand, ready to lift your knees, one at a time.
- Lift your right hand into the air and slap your left knee as you let out a big cowboy. Yee-Haw and laugh!
- Lift your left hand into the air and slap your right knee as you let out a big cowboy Yee-Haw and laugh!
- Repeat three to five times.

Extra: Greet each other every day with a "Very good! Very good! Yay!" or greet them with a "Yay!" or a "Whoo Hoo!" Say anything other than "How are you?" You can also extend your goodbyes for the day with the same or other made-up good night greetings. And always add a smile or laughter!

"If laughter cannot solve your problems, it will definitely dissolve them by changing your body chemistry and mindset so you can face them in a better way." ~ Dr. Madan Kataria

Personal Note

I have been doing Laughter Yoga for 15 minutes per day (plus the classes I teach) for five and a half years. I have never been this happy—ever. It's mind-blowing! Not only have I become aware of stress and its effects on me physically, mentally and emotionally, but it has also provided me with a vehicle to stop excess cortisol and enter into the magical realm of the Blue Road and the happiness hormones.

Most importantly, I was in a devastating car accident twenty-two months ago. My ND/Iridologist/Herbalist provided my most important holistic healthcare. I followed all her recommendations, and my body has done major healing, slowly but surely. During this time, I did at least fifteen minutes of Laughter Yoga per day, fifteen minutes of Tibetan Humming and (later) added 15 minutes of HeartMath Coherence Breathing. Last January, my holistic practitioner shared with me that she never thought I would rehab to the degree that I have! During these long months, the only pain reliever I took was occasional aspirin, and my inner and outer injuries have healed beyond belief. I have only minor lower back pain and some knee pain left. I attribute my remarkable pain relief/healing to Laughter Yoga. I am grateful! I live in gratitude in knowing how to access the Blue Road "slice of heaven" at any time. And, I am joyous of my glowing eyes and the Mona Lisa smile that my face often displays.

Exciting News

The Laughter Yoga International Organization, headed by Dr. Madan Kataria, is awaiting final approval to present one minute of Laughter Yoga during the Opening Ceremonies of the 2020 Olympics in Japan. This is a big deal! Can you imagine all the good vibes that will be created as millions of people around the world laugh together—all at the same time—for world peace? Wow! For information on Laughter Yoga, go to LaughterYoga.org.

An Invitation

I am interested in what people who travel from the Red Road to the Blue Road experience. If you would like to share your experiences with me please contact me.

CHAPTER

Ten

Path To Peace
By Jill Tyge

JILL TYGE

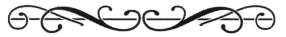

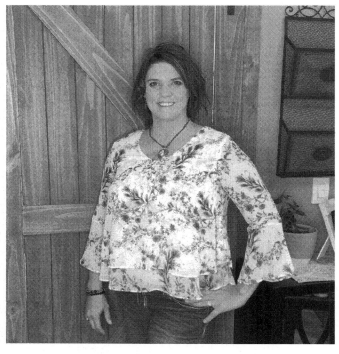

Jill Tyge is a mind, body, spirit practitioner specializing in healing trauma in families and homes. As an Awakening Your Light Body meditation guide, Trailblazing Communication practitioner, and owner of Pura Vida Peace, LLC., she has been on a mission to help women take back their power, heal from loss or abuse, shift energy from family trauma, and create balance in their lives with her many healing modalities including meditation, energy work, and using her intuition. Jill is available to travel and provide tools and support to women who are ready to improve their daily lives and environment. When not working, Jill enjoys traveling, spending time with family, being outdoors, sitting around a fire or by the water, hiking, watching football and hockey, reading, and adding new tools to her tool belt. Email: jilltyge@gmail.com; Facebook: www.facebook.com/puravidapeace; Website: www.jilltyge.com

Acknowledgments

I would like to thank my husband, Jason—my best friend, my rock—encouraging me to chase my dreams. You stepped in, becoming our biggest supporter and cheerleader. We are lucky and blessed to share life with you. To my children, who always guide me to what I need to explore further, and make me aware when we are off-balance. You are such a blessing. I am proud to be your mom. To Wes Hamilton, for teaching me the amazing gift of meditation, I admire and appreciate your guidance. To Tara Argall, your amazing gifts and talents by developing energy tools to help us heal ourselves. To Shanda Trofe and Carrie Severson, for helping find my voice, my story, and the courage to use them. I am truly grateful. Finally, my guides, God, spirits, angels, and all who have been there to guide and support my journey. Thank you!

Path To Peace
By Jill Tyge

My healing journey began in 2009, while I was a mom to three little kids, worked full-time, and was a wife to someone who was hardly around. Though I was extremely busy, I was far from fulfilled. In fact, I was barely existing as I went through the motions, doing the same thing day in and day out as I tried to keep the house together. Then one night as I was working, my husband walked into my home office and said, "This is what you are going to amount to in life?"

His words shook me to the core, and not just because they were cruel or because he didn't seem to notice that I was exhausted from doing everything, without much help from him, to make our family work. I had often had the same thoughts that I wanted more out of life and that I wanted to feel like I meant more. I wanted to be appreciated for what I was doing. I wanted joy and happiness. I wanted a purpose. That night was my wakeup call. It was time for change. It was time for me to grow and find my individual path. It was time to start exploring.

The first class I took was an Awakening Your Light Body meditation class, which met one Saturday a month for six months. Each class, we would get a new set of twelve meditations that we would spend the next month working on. Here is a brief description of what occurred and can occur while being guided by these meditations, as explained and described by DaBen and Orin.

The process begins with building your power base, which helps you remain calm and centered around other people's energy and changes your emotional and personality reactions to others. It also helps you to be transparent to lower energies. It helps evolve your inner child, release and transform old habits and patterns, and work with various parts of your personality to prepare for the rapid growth that can occur as you awaken your light body.

The second part is opening the heart center. This creates flow and assists you in experiencing love. This center will awaken your inner healer and help you learn about self-healing. You will also discover ways to stay neutral around others and create greater physical vitality.

Part three of the series is working with your higher energy centers. This helps a person to experience their higher mind and increases both their creativity and their ability to find creative solutions to challenges. It also helps you experience higher, more positive and unlimited thoughts, and to manifest what you want for your higher purpose in life.

The fourth part is aligning with vibrational energy bodies. This makes you aware of subtle, higher energies and to make these energies a part of your life and consciousness. You will be able to quiet your thoughts, feel energized, and enhance your inner vision and intuitive abilities. You will also recharge your energy at the core, feel harmonized and balanced, and transform relationships and abundance issues by working on them first as energy, then being open to experience the changes that can occur. Perhaps most importantly, you will learn how to choose the way you want to feel.

The fifth part is awakening your light body. Here, you will start to experience states of joy, inner visualizations, feelings, and sensations that are beautiful beyond words. You will learn how to connect soul-to-soul with loved ones to transform your relationships and to radiate light to others. You will learn to become a breath with the Universe, journey into oneness, and learn how to exist in this dimension while remaining aware of other dimensions. You will clear, purify, and add higher frequencies to your aura. You will learn how to become a source of light.

Finally, the last part is becoming radiant. This opens you to experience incredible bliss and beauty. It connects you directly with the light, brings in the light from higher dimensions, and regulates, filters, and integrates light as you bring it in. You will work with your personality to help it hold, in a balanced way, the enormity of the perspective you are gaining with regard to your soul, your purpose, and the insights you may have as you experience the Universe in new ways.

This class certainly shifted my perspective. As my soul found its voice, it continued to take me to various different classes, experiences, and teachers. As I continued to grow and expand, I noticed the effect it was having on others in my life, including my children. I learned that when we take care of ourselves and raise our vibration, it slowly brings up the vibration of the entire house and the people living in it. If the people in the house don't like the change in vibration, they will fall away. Children, in particular, are our mirrors, reflecting where we are in any particular moment. Energy affects the entire family, including the relationships we have with each other and our financial abundance. That said, children do carry some ancestral patterns and traumas that have been passed down through the generations, built into their DNA and subconscious. I learned that we need to heal ourselves, and the effects of this healing will ripple out to our children. Most importantly, I learned that we all must take ownership of our lives and accountability for our choices, for only then can we step into our power as the creators we truly are.

My inner work also began to play out in my marriage, though not in a way I would have anticipated. The more I worked on myself and made choices that would empower me to grow and learn, the unhappier my husband was, and the more volatile our relationship became. We tried counseling for months, but it didn't get us anywhere. It got to the point where I didn't know what the truth was anymore. I filed for divorce after I was thrown across the living room onto the couch in front of two of my children. I thought that leaving the marriage would make my life better, that I would be able to do what I wanted and would be happier. Unfortunately, that was only the beginning of the hardest journey I have had to walk, but it also has given me lots of tools, confidence, and a new approach to how I do life.

It took me a while to understand how toxic my marriage was. One day in mediation, a lawyer told me she would no longer work with us. She also told me to go look up narcissism and said that in twenty-two years of practicing law, my soon-to-be-ex was one of the most difficult she had ever seen. I read and studied as much as I could about the subject and found my best resource was Shahida Arabi's, *Becoming the Narcissist's Nightmare: How to Devalue and Discard the Narcissist While Supplying Yourself.*

Arabi best explains narcissistic abuse as the chronic manipulation and devaluation of their victims, leaving them feeling worthless, anxious, and even suicidal. This type of continual manipulation includes idealization-devaluation-discard abuse cycle where they "love-bomb" their partners, devalue them, then discard them until the trauma begins again. Other toxic behaviors associated with this type of abuse can include, but are not limited to, being overly critical and controlling, and covertly and overtly putting victims down through verbal abuse and manipulative behaviors that are intended to isolate and demean them. Narcissists are all about using contempt for others as a way to demonstrate their power and gain a false sense of superiority. They manufacture hostile or aggressive situations in which the victim is led to emotional distress, and create environments where the victim feels trapped, controlled, and limited in what he or she can say or do. They gradually control every aspect of the victim's life, to the point of isolating them from friends and family and sabotaging important life events, goals, and aspirations. If the victim voices concerns about the relationship, the narcissist will stonewall them into silence, deny, minimalize or rationalize the abuse, engage in pathological lying and deceit, and subject the victims to smear campaigns to make him/her look like the "crazy one."

As I read this book, I cried and cried. Arabi was describing my life. It was what I was living day by day. Even after I left the marriage, I was living in constant fear. There were times when I didn't feel safe in my house. I tried to distance myself by moving an hour away, but my ex followed, although it lengthened his commute to work. Every time I tried to move forward and do something new and better with my life, he would do something to try to push it off course. When I tried to have a new relationship, he moved in across the street. He also kept changing our schedule with the kids, so it was difficult for me to make plans. If I made plans to be out of town while he had the kids, he would no-show or call the night before (or on his way to the airport!) to tell me that he would not be around. If I said no to a schedule change, he would find a way to retaliate, even to the point of sneaking the kids out of school, and out of town, without my knowledge. I didn't know where they were or when they would be back.

He loved to go to lawyers and judges to get things in writing and make himself look powerful. I told these legal experts what he was doing—I even had the patterns documented—but no one would listen to me. When he snuck the kids out of town, the judge's answer was for me to come back to court. Why bother, I thought, when he has never been held accountable for anything except child support? In the meantime, I was losing friends, family, and the support of the people who would help me with the children.

This went on for a number of years. My ex-husband would not accept the boundaries I set up. I was constantly being watched, and often walking on eggshells afraid of what was going to happen next. The worst part has been watching my children go through it. Oftentimes, I think it is harder than when I was living it myself. He doesn't realize the effect his games and manipulation has on them, and what it can do to them down the road. Through my inner work, I have realized that this is the kids' lesson to learn. I can't control their journey or the path they need to take. All I can do is provide them with the tools to transmute the trauma and heal themselves when they are ready.

When I realized what I was living through, I started to heal myself through meditation, body talk, dowsing, and reading books about healing from trauma, while going to lectures on different ways to heal. When I needed help, I asked for it, including from a friend of mine who years earlier had used body talk on my children to help them shift the trauma of the divorce. Later, when one of my children was struggling in school, I reached out to her again. We met, and she shared with me an energy program she had developed called Trailblazing Communications. It was a program that could be used on people, animals, businesses, homes, land, and nutrition. It was also a way for the non-verbal to communicate.

She did a session for my son and yielded excellent results in a short amount of time. I signed up for the classes and the program so I could use it on a regular basis on myself and others. I check in almost every day to raise the vibration, make sure we are protected, and see if any sessions are needed for the day. If I go a week or two without doing sessions or keeping up the family's energy (usually when we're on vacation), it will show up in our lives as complete and utter chaos, and I immediately resume my practice to get things back into balance.

"Pain travels through family lines until someone is ready to heal it in themselves. By going through the agony of healing, you no longer pass the poison chalice onto the generations that follow. It is incredibly important and sacred work." ~ Unknown

We have a lot of broken systems in place right now, things that perhaps were helpful at one time but for many no longer work. We need to go to the root and heal the trauma we may have experienced growing up, or we will have children who continue to this pass on. Going within ourselves will help us understand and heal. People who have lived through a lot of trauma don't feel bad about how they treat others; instead, they often lie and manipulate others to get what they want because this is how they learned to survive. They usually have not been held accountable and don't have feelings about how they behave, or what they are doing to someone else's reputation or wellbeing. Trailblazing has helped me shift family patterns and traumas so they will not continue to be passed down to future generations.

Sometimes the way we help and shift has to be in an unconventional way. The work that I have done on myself and my children has time and again validated my ability to clear patterns, shift the energy, and heal us. Have we had bumps in the road? Have I made mistakes along the way? Yes—mistakes are how we change and grow. I have been alone in my journey, and I now am okay with that. I want other women in my situation to know that we can thrive from this. We can all make a difference in the world and help our kids. We must realize, however, that this sometimes means letting go and understanding that it is their journey, and they will make the choices they need to make to learn and grow.

It has been a rocky road that I have walked, many times questioning my every turn or roadblock. My goal has always been, and continues to be, to be the best I can be, to be the best mom, and the most authentic me. Have I met predators along the way who have made me fight back? You bet. But then I recoil back into myself and either learn and grow or head down a different path. There have been many teachers and lessons along the way, but the best tools I have are meditation, which gives me the clarity, the insight, and the answers, and Trailblazing, which helps me shift the energy, the pattern, and the result. These tools have been my road-map and compass, and they are always in my bag as I hop in the car and head down the path to freedom. If you need a tour guide to help you find your path to healing, I would love to walk beside you, help you find your path, and let you know you are not alone. Safe travels and happy shifting to a beautiful life!

CHAPTER

Eleven

Let Your Superpower Flow
By Dr. JuJu Love

DR. JUJU LOVE

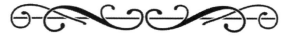

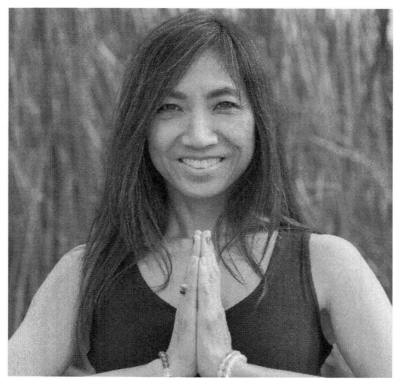

Dr. JuJu Love is a transformative holistic wellness goddess. Prior to her career in the wellness industry, she served as an art director in New York City for over a decade. When the company was acquired by a consumer market giant, she opted to take the opportunity to walk away and pursue her quest for self-discovery in full force. During her journey of self-discovery, she experienced a spiritual awakening that transformed her life into that of a healer in service to humanity. She's been walking the path of a holistic healer for the past 15 years, and along her journey, she also became a licensed naturopathic doctor in the state of Arizona. Her passion is to guide people to their soul/spiritual awakening so they can live the life they are meant to have with love, peace, joy, and harmony. DrJuJuLove.com, drjujulove888@gmail.com, 646-734-7304.

Acknowledgments

My heartfelt thanks and deepest appreciation to my friends, family, my inner goddess, and the divine guidance from the source and many beings of divine love and light.

Let Your Superpower Flow
By Dr. JuJu Love

"I slept and dreamt that life was joy. I awoke and saw that
life was service. I acted and behold, service was joy."
~ Rabindranath Tagore

One thing I am sure about life at this tender age of 54,
is that it never ceases to amaze me for it fills me up
with constant wonder and awe. Life sometimes
throws a curveball at you when you least expect it and puts
you on a path you've never imagined for yourself. I am
blessed to have received some of those magical curveballs in
my life, and each time it put me on a completely different
path than the one I thought I was supposed to take, and I am
forever grateful.

The Beginning

"Ask, and it will be given to you; search, and you will find;
knock, and the door will be opened for you. For everyone
who asks receives, and everyone who searches finds, and
for everyone who knocks, the door will be opened."
~ Matthew 7:7-8

The first magical curveball came at me when I was 15
years old, and transplanted me from Korea to America. It
opened my eyes to a whole new world, helped me learn a
new language and new skills, find new friends, and develop
new awareness of diversities in people and culture that I
hadn't experienced while growing up in Korea. It also made

me aware that I felt more at home in this new land than in my homeland.

Another magical curveball came in my mid-thirties, when I thought I had my life all figured out with a seemingly happy marriage, a great job as an art director in New York City, a pretty house, and money being no object. However, I felt something was amiss, and the feelings of a deep void inside were seeping into every aspect of my life. On an unassuming Saturday afternoon, I was catapulted into witnessing the last moment of my life. Suffice it to say I was shocked by what I witnessed, because I realized that I had never lived, and my life was about to expire. I had mind-lessly wasted my entire life, and my existence had no meaning. When I came out of the trance, I was depressed because my existence made no sense to me. This was the beginning of my deep self-inquiry and spiritual journey, asking who am I, what's my purpose, what's my passion, and what's the meaning of life for me? A series of syn-chronous events eventually led me to experience the most profound transformative spiritual awakening and activation of the gift of healing from the universe. From that time on, my inner healer, goddess, teacher, and artist have been guiding me not only through my healing journey, but also the healing journeys of countless others.

Wounded Healer

"Only the wounded physician heals." ~ Carl Jung

Following my awakening was an intense period of what I refer to as my *quickening*. During this time, I was overflowing with love and joy and feeling ecstatic and intoxicated with divine love. Healing came to me naturally and intuitively and was effortless because all I had to do was step aside and observe while a divine, angelic, feminine being would step into my place and orchestrate it. Sometimes, working on someone was like watching a play with a lot of actors on the stage of body and energy fields. These actors were animated, emotionally charged, and often in conflict with one another. I wanted to know who these actors were, but I didn't know the first thing about human anatomy, so I was left clueless. At that time, the Universe introduced to me the BodyTalk System, a form of energy medicine founded by Dr. John Veltheim. Since the body was already talking to me in cryptic messages, the name of this modality piqued my interest. I received a Bodytalk session from the acupuncturist who introduced me to it, and I signed up to learn about it the first chance I had. It was fascinating to learn how this simple, elegant modality navigates the complex body-mind-spirit connection. I quickly became a certified BodyTalker, and added to my growing repertoire of healing tools.

As I saturated myself in the beautiful healing energy that I associated with divine love, I found joy and passion in the healing arts and being in service to others in their healing journeys. I set up a holistic healing practice and started seeing clients. Although each client had unique ailments and challenges, I made an interesting discovery. Most of them suffered from anxiety and depression. Another thing I noticed was they were highly sensitive, deeply caring, and empathic. They all seemed to reflect back to me parts of my struggles, because being an empath with heightened sensitivity, I used to suffer from some levels of anxiety and depression, frequent migraines and gastrointestinal (GI) issues, commonly known as irritable bowel syndrome (IBS), premenstrual syndromes (PMS), an addictive behavior as a cigarette smoker, and an eating disorder, specifically, bulimia. Working with these people taught me more about myself and helped me better understand my challenges. It was as if the Universe was bringing these people to me deliberately so I could learn and explore the relationship between these common traits and their health and well-being while healing myself.

Expansion as a Doctor Who is a Healer

"Emotions are at the nexus between mind and matter, going back and forth between the two and influencing both."
~ Candace Pert, *Molecules of Emotions*

My continuing desire to serve led me to further investigate Ayurveda, acupuncture, massage therapy, psychoanalysis, and nutrition. I found them to be great healing arts, and would support them whole-heartedly, but none of them spoke to my heart enough to pursue. In the meantime, my wanting to learn more of the human anatomy and physiology led me to discover Naturopathic Medicine, and I instantly fell in love with their principles.

The fundamental principles of Naturopathic Medicine:

1. First, do no harm (*Primum non nocere*)
   - Choose the most non-invasive and least toxic treatments necessary.
2. The healing power of nature (*Vis medicatrix naturae*)
   - Utilize the body's inherent ability to heal itself.
3. Identify and treat the causes (*Tolle causam*)

- Identify, address, and remove the underlying causes of disease.
4. Doctor as teacher (*Docere*)
   - Educating and empowering patients to take responsibility for their health.
5. Treat the whole person (*Tolle totum*)
   - The body as an integrated whole. Treat the patient, not the disease. Address the nutritional status, lifestyle, family history, physical, mental, emotional, genetic, environmental, and social factors in a person's life.
6. Prevention (*Praevenic*)
   - Focus on overall health, wellness, and disease prevention.

Southwest College of Naturopathic Medicine in Arizona was the school of my choice because acupuncture and traditional Chinese medicine were part of the program, which also includes biomedical sciences, nutrition, botanical medicine, environmental medicine, homeopathic medicine, psychology, counseling, minor surgery, and women's medicine. Without hesitation, I uprooted myself from New York, where I had lived for nearly three decades, and moved to Arizona, where I didn't know a soul, in pursuit of becoming a naturopathic physician. Looking back, I wonder if I would have gone through the program had I known how difficult it was going to be. But the fact is that I didn't, so I put my head down and plowed through the program because there was no Option B for me!

After passing the licensing board exams, I started my practice as a naturopathic physician. I noticed similar patterns in my patient population, such as anxiety, depression, and hypersensitivity, plus varying degrees of other chronic symptoms, such as chronic migraines, frequent headaches, IBS and gastrointestinal issues, chronic fatigue, thyroid conditions, PMS, sleep issues, adrenal burnout, backaches and joint pains, hormonal imbalances, metabolic dysfunction, and autoimmune conditions including fibromyalgia, rheumatoid arthritis, and Hashimoto's thyroiditis.

This time, I felt better equipped to guide my patients in their healing journeys because I've healed quite a few of my personal challenges and am still improving. Moreover, I've become familiar with Dr. Elaine Aron's work on the Highly Sensitive Person (HSP), and have a better understanding of the biochemical and physiological implications stress has on the body, how emotions affect our physiology and the power of our mindset.

Let the Healing Begin

"You are not broken. You are not crazy. You are exactly who you are meant to be, a super-sensitive being. It is your superpower. As you cultivate it and learn how to navigate it better, you will see that it's your divine gift and blessing, not something you need to fix or avoid." ~ Dr. JuJu Love

First, let's talk about HSPs. According to research by Elaine Aron, high sensitivity is an innate trait that is often inherited and found in 15-20 percent of the population. This trait allows the nervous system and brain to process subtleties in the surroundings that others miss. However, HSPs become easily burdened by overstimulation from prolonged exposures to high stimuli in the environment. She says there are two classes of people, the aggressive warrior-kings who thrive on expansion, freedom, and fame, and the thoughtful royal advisors who direct the wonderful expansive energy of the society from aggression and domination, and use it for the highest good of all. She says HSPs are the royal advisors who are creative types, artists, philosophers, teachers, researchers, theologians, therapist, historians, and conscientious members of the earth.

Can you identify yourself with any of the challenges and strengths of HSPs?

Common HSP challenges:

• Anxiety and depression

• Nervous and emotional exhaustion from sensory overload

• Overwhelm causing anxiety, chronic digestive issues, fatigue, brain fog, lowered immunity

• Heightened sensitivity to pain

• Easily startled

• Intense emotions, both positive and negative, and sensitivity to others' emotions

• Shyness

• Social anxiety

• Low self-esteem

• Feeling misunderstood

• Boundary issues

• Conflict avoidance

• Difficulty making quick decisions

• Difficulty with changes

• Delayed milestones

• Tendency to self-sacrifice

HSP strengths:

• Empathetic

• Intuitive

• Perceptive

• Creative

• Feel deeply

• Think deeply

• Seeker

• Aware of subtleties

• Conscientious

• Love nature and animals

• Despise violence and cruelty

Many of you are already aware that stress is the main culprit to declining health and wellness. Stress can come from many sources; physical, environmental, and emotional. As I mentioned, being an HSP has the challenge of feeling everything more intensely than the rest, which can be overwhelming to the body and mind. Your nervous system can be frazzled, and if it goes unchecked, it will cause stress that can manifest as real health issues.

According to Dr. Hans Selye, the biology of stress mainly affects three types of tissues/organs in the body; the adrenal glands in the hormonal system; the spleen, the thymus and the lymph glands in the immune system; and the lining of the intestines in the digestive system. You may be able to see how constant overstimulation of HSPs nervous systems can affect their health over time. It may show up as adrenal fatigue, sleep issues, overproduction of stress hormone leading to osteoporosis and intestinal ulcers, other hormonal imbalances, frequent colds and flu, and allergies due to lowered immune function. Selye says the most important stressors for man are emotional.

Anxiety and depression are common symptoms among HSPs, especially with a lack of secure bonding during childhood and meaningful adult relationships. In *The Biology of Belief*, Dr. Bruce Lipton explains that chronically stressful events in early childhood get programmed into the nervous system, operating under the influence of the brain's emotional centers. They become the cellular memory of the unconscious beliefs that override your conscious thoughts and control what you feel and how you react to events later on. These unconscious beliefs can produce enough stress to cause many disease processes. For healing to take place, the biology of belief adopted early in life needs to be undone. Healing is a dynamic interplay between the mind, body, and spirit. It's not a static or one-directional thing; it's an inside job.

We all have challenges and struggles. No one is exempt from them because only through them do we truly evolve to unfold the higher potential we possess. It is a lifelong process. We never truly arrive at one particular place in life to stay there, but journey through it. The beauty is in the journey, and joy is in witnessing and experiencing it fully with open arms and heart. It's up to you what you do with the gifts the Universe blesses you with. You can choose to fight and struggle with them or learn how to wield them to create what you want in life.

Activate Your Inner Healer!

If you are an HSP, it's imperative you take time for yourself regularly and de-stress. It's not being selfish. It's self-care to show self-love!

Healing Tool Chest – Dr. JuJu Love Recommends:

- Labs
  - o To check for any imbalances in blood and hormones, or other underlying causes such as viral or bacterial infections, autoimmunity, food sensitivities, and environmental toxicities.

- Basic supplements and nutrients, which I take and recommend to my clients
  - o Fish oil
  - o Vitamin B complex
  - o Magnesium
  - o Probiotics
  - o Vitamin C
  - o Vitamin D & K
  - o L-Glutamine for GI issues or ulcer
  - o Ashwagandha for fatigue or difficulty sleeping
- Diet Nutrition
  - o Minimize processed sugar consumption.
  - o Avoid food sensitivity foods (if you don't know where to start: sugar, wheat, soy, corn, dairy, eggs, shellfish, peanuts).

- o Avoid GMOs.
- o Organic foods whenever possible.
- o Apple cider vinegar.
- o Dark leafy greens.
- o Cruciferous vegetables (broccoli, kale, cauliflower, brussels sprouts, cabbage).
- o Good fat.
- o Plenty of pure water.
- o Avoid stimulants like caffeine.
- Daily positive mindset practice.
  - o Self-inquiry—ask yourself the following questions when an unpleasant negative emotion surfaces:
    - ▪ "Is it true?"
    - ▪ "Who would I be without ___?"
    - ▪ "How is it serving me?"
  - o Affirmations – keep them positive without using negating words.
  - o Gratitude journal—write down 10 things, morning and night.
  - o "I am" declaration – make a list of your "I am" declarations and read them out loud three times, morning and night.
- Mindfulness practice
  - o Meditation—either sit with your back straight or lay down, focus on your breath, and chant "om," or do it your preferred way.
- Visualization
  - o Visualize a healing light of the color and shape of your choice transmuting any pains

or health issues you have in your body, and challenges in your life.

- Breathwork
  - o Breath is life. Use it to move energy, restore calmness, and clear energy blocks and stuck emotions.
  - o Engage your diaphragm when you breathe. Put one of your hands on your solar plexus. Your hand should come out with each inhalation, and go in with each exhalation.
  - o Breathe rhythmically, slowly and calmly without stressing.
- Move your body! Exercise, martial arts, Qi Gong, yoga, and dance.
- Sing! It opens up your throat chakra, your self-expression center.
- Create art. Draw, paint, get your hands dirty and make something. Exercise your creator essence.
- Spend time in nature and walk barefoot. Unplug from the artificial world and plug into Gaia.
- Receive regular energy healing, reiki, bodywork, and massages.
- Do Emotional Freedom Technique (EFT)—tapping to shift any unconscious beliefs.
- Give and receive hugs whenever you can. It activates the love hormone, oxytocin.
- Laugh often, it activates endorphins. It's the best form of stress management and it's completely free!

CHAPTER

Twelve

The Unseen Therapist
By Karen Gabler

KAREN GABLER

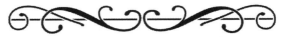

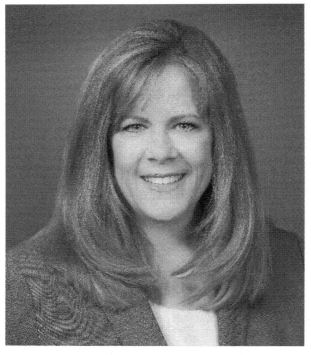

Karen Gabler is an attorney, intuitive coach, and psychic medium. She is also a published author and inspirational speaker. Karen is passionate about encouraging others to live their best lives. She provides her clients with intuitive information and guidance regarding their personal and business questions and facilitates connections with their loved ones in spirit. Karen also conducts seminars and workshops on a variety of spiritual, business, and personal development topics. Karen earned her Bachelor of Science in psychology and her Juris Doctorate from the University of Hawaii. She has pursued wide-ranging education in interpersonal development and the spiritual sciences, working with tutors from the prestigious Arthur Findlay College for the Psychic Sciences in England, as well as with intuitive coaches and psychic mediums throughout the United States. She enjoys reading, horseback riding, and spending time with her husband and two children. You can find Karen at www.karengabler.com.

Acknowledgments

"At times, our light goes out and is rekindled by a spark from another person. Each of us has cause to think with deep gratitude of those who have lighted the flame within us." ~ Albert Schweitzer.

I'd like to give a special thanks to my family and friends who have supported me on my path to finding and living my inner truth, so that I could in turn fully express my desire and ability to help others do the same in more ways than I ever thought possible. When I shine, it is with your light inside me. Each of you has rekindled my spark and lit the flame within me in your individual way, some of you many times over, and I am eternally grateful for it and for you.

The Unseen Therapist
By Karen Gabler

You once told me
You wanted to find
Yourself in the world—
And I told you to
First, apply within,
To discover the world within you.

We are quick to look outside ourselves for answers to the questions that lie within us. We scroll social media sites, wondering why everyone else's lives seem so much more vibrant than ours. We try the latest diet; we read the latest self-help book. We watch reality television, holding it up as a mirror to ourselves.

In fact, we came here with all the answers stored inside us. We are spiritual beings, exploring a human existence. Like a new computer that comes pre-loaded with critical software, we need only activate the programming embedded within our souls to find our way back to each other and ourselves.

There are a variety of ways to connect with our inner selves, many of which can be achieved individually. Meditation, journaling, spending time in nature, and similar tools can help us to connect, clearing away outside noise and activating the guidance within. At times, however, our human ego drowns out the subtle soul guidance. We second-guess our intuitive knowledge and question whether we are "making it up."

Intuitive coaches, mediums and psychics can provide a better understanding of when our human is speaking to us and when we are actually hearing from our soul, a loved one in spirit, or a source of higher knowledge. Working with an intuitive professional can jump-start our intuition, ensuring that we look to our inner guidance systems for the answers we desire.

Accessing honest and ethical professional support requires an understanding of the intuitive process and a level of discernment as to whether the messages you are receiving are genuinely coming from the right place. Spiritual guidance should never reprimand, frighten, burden or limit you. Instead, intuitive messages should always serve your highest good and provide insights of love, hope, and healing.

Mediumship

"Mark" requested a mediumship reading to connect with his loved ones in spirit. As we began the reading, I became aware of a man who felt like Mark's father. He appeared with a tulip, holding it out to the woman next to him who identified herself as Mark's mother. The father held out a briefcase. The mother said, "Don't drop the baby!" They showed me a newborn child, swaddled in a yellow blanket with a brown duck. They made me aware of a family party coming up and said they intended to be there.

Mark confirmed that his parents were in spirit. He shared that his father often surprised his mother with tulips, her favorite flower. Mark relayed that his father was an obstetrician. He carried his brown briefcase to work every day; Mark's mother would kiss him goodbye and say, "Don't drop the babies!" as he left the house. Mark had tears in his eyes as he relayed that his daughter was born six months earlier, and he had wondered if his parents knew she had arrived. He shook his head in disbelief as he shared that he had brought his daughter home from the hospital in a yellow blanket with a duck embroidered on it.

Mark said the only thing he couldn't place was the family party; there was no such party planned. On his way home, Mark called his sister to share his mediumship experience. She told him she was glad he called because she was talking with her husband about planning a family reunion that summer and wanted to tell Mark about her plans. Stunned, Mark laughed as he told her that their parents were planning to attend the party.

When our loved ones pass to spirit, they are truly only a thought away. Spirits communicate energetically, impressing thoughts, feelings and images upon the medium. A medium is a translator, turning vibrational communication from discarnate spirits into information recognizable to the client. Some mediums describe it as translating a spoken language—if your family member spoke a different language, wouldn't it make sense to find a translator to facilitate your conversation?

Our loved ones want us to know that they are still around us. We may wonder if they are still in pain or whether they suffered in their transition. We may want to know what they see of our lives after they are gone. Understanding that a loved one is safe and happy can relieve our concerns, and learning that they are still present in our lives can make us feel less alone.

Mediumship also may provide much-needed healing. If we have experienced painful relationships with others, their death may deny us satisfactory closure. Whether or not we are ready to forgive those who wronged us in life, their acknowledgment of their behavior can release us to move forward. Recognizing that our loved ones can communicate with us also can begin to answer our questions about what will happen to us when we leave this earth.

To have the best mediumistic experience, invite your loved ones to the session. Consider bringing relevant photos, jewelry, or other items with you. You may hope to hear from a particular person or receive a specific message, but remain open to anyone and anything that comes through. There are many reasons why a particular person may not appear. Energetic communication is a skill on both sides, and some spirits are more apt to step forward than others, especially if they did so in life. Your loved one may not resonate with this particular medium, or the medium may more easily recognize personalities that feel familiar to them. It is never because a spirit doesn't want to talk to you, nor have you done anything wrong.

You should never be asked (nor should you volunteer) to provide detailed factual information to the medium; this may cause you to question whether it was "real." Recognize that mediums are human, and may misinterpret information. Like a spiritual game of "telephone," the message conveyed may not be quite what the spirit intended. When you verify accurate information and reject incorrect information, the medium can ask the spirit for help to correct any misstatements.

Most of all, remember that your loved ones will not tell you what to do, nor will they reprimand or argue with you. They retain the same personality they exhibited in life, but will typically demonstrate a greater understanding of themselves and others (or acknowledge that they are working on it). Mediumship readings should provide a connection with your loved ones and a healing opportunity. Work only with mediums who are open and honest about the process, operate from a place of service rather than ego, and demonstrate love and respect for the spirit world.

Psychic (Soul) Readings

"Laurie" entered the room with a look of despair. Her marriage was faltering. She relayed that while working with a life coach, she had discussed her husband's seeming disinterest in her or their lives together. Her coach encouraged her to find strength within herself and move on to begin a new life without him.

As I connected with her, I received the clear message that there was a great deal of love remaining in her marriage. I could feel that she and her husband stood silently together, but each looked outward at the world rather than toward each other. In this vision, I could see them turn toward each other, join hands, and step outside to face the world together. I received multiple messages about where they had veered off track and how they could reconnect.

Laurie broke down in tears. She said, "I felt so awful when my coach told me that my marriage was over. I didn't want to be done, but she told me that I was hanging on to the past." I shared that she and her husband may have lost their way, but there was lots to explore before giving up. They had forgotten to have fun together and needed to revisit some of the activities they used to enjoy as a couple before starting a family. I became aware of the weekend trips they had taken and their shared love of the theater. I could also feel that Laurie's husband had even less confidence in their relationship than she did, and I let her know that it might take several attempts to encourage him to explore their relationship once again.

Laurie later contacted me to let me know that she had acted on the guidance she received in her reading, and that she and her husband were taking tentative steps toward each other once again. While they weren't completely "out of the woods," she knew that whether or not it worked out, she would feel confident that they had given their relationship everything they could, and everything it deserved.

In our day-to-day lives, we forget why we are here, what we are meant to do, and who we genuinely are. Although we receive a constant stream of intuitive "hits," we may fail to notice or accept that information. A psychic reading can access what your soul wants your human to know about your life path. It can reconnect you to yourself in a profound way, allowing you to recognize and trust the information you have been receiving all along. When your soul communicates with you, it does so with love, support, and a desire for your highest and best good.

Psychics are not fortune-tellers and cannot predict the future. We all have free will and our future changes from minute to minute, based upon the myriad of choices we make each day. Our lives are like a tree with many branches. A prediction is a snapshot in time—this is what could happen if absolutely nothing changes for you after the reading. Naturally, this is impossible. When we move in a new direction, we flutter to another branch on our tree. New branches sprout all the time, and the possibilities that lie before us are endless.

To experience the best possible psychic reading, set your intention to receive guidance for your highest and best good. Jot down any questions; you may find that your questions are answered during the reading without even asking. Disregard any message that makes you feel insecure, frightened, sad, or upset in any way, while remaining open to information you may not have considered before. Again, work with an intuitive professional who comes from a place of service rather than ego, and who treats both your human self and your soul self with the utmost respect.

Intuitive Coaching

"Victoria" was invited to speak at a conference in Denver. Her involvement would include national publication of her photos and participation in radio interviews. She knew this would be a giant step forward in her career, and told herself to feel grateful for the opportunity. And yet, something inside her was ringing alarm bells—she knew that this could be a serious mistake.

Victoria reached out for an intuitive coaching session to better understand whether she should listen to her intuition and skip the conference, or whether she was blocking her personal success with irrational fears. We discussed her hesitations. In connecting with her guides and helpers, in spirit, I became aware that her fears were connected to her mother, and we began exploring early messages she might have received about shining in the world.

After initially questioning why I would bring up her mother in a conversation about the conference, Victoria recalled that her mother was attacked by a man masquerading as a business client when Victoria was a young girl. In recovering from this painful incident, Victoria's mother admonished her five-year-old daughter that safety required protecting yourself and your identity. Exposing your name and photo to the world would put you at risk, and playing on a national stage would be inviting tragedy. As this information came up, Victoria expressed shock, exclaiming, "I didn't even remember that we ever talked about that. She never wanted to discuss it; it never occurred to me that I carried it with me."

By combining intuitive guidance with Victoria's memories, we were able to separate Victoria's limiting beliefs, received from a well-intentioned parent at a tender age, from the reality of the conference opportunity. Receiving intuitive guidance about what to ask and how to help her in our session allowed the coaching process to move forward quickly; we rapidly accessed information that Victoria would not have considered without gentle prodding from a higher source. Victoria enthusiastically accepted the conference invitation, requesting reasonable limits around her published information. She contacted me later to share that the conference was an exceptional success, resulting in new clients and speaking opportunities and increased confidence in herself.

It is common for our personal stories and limiting beliefs to interfere with our life path, often without our awareness that it is occurring. Even when we know that we feel blocked, we may not know why. Our success depends upon reframing those stories and clearing those blocks. Intuitive coaching can streamline the process of doing so by accessing not only the information provided (directly or indirectly) by the client, but also through other intuitive sources.

We come here with spiritual guides to support us on our path. We all have equal access to higher knowledge and support obtained through a variety of sources, including teachers, healers, ascended masters, angels and archangels, God (as defined by us), and the Universe itself. They provide constant information and support, accessible to us at any time. They also course-correct when we veer off our path, gently steering us back to our true life purpose.

An intuitive coach is a mirror, guiding you to know and do what you came here knowing how to do but have forgotten along the way. An intuitive coach teaches you to access and trust your intuition and universal guidance, allowing you to identify the blocks that prevent you from achieving your life purpose and understanding the steps necessary to progress. Intuitive coaching brings your innate needs, desires, and purpose to the surface, and clears away anything that limits you in living your highest and best life.

Although we carry all that we need within us and can connect to our souls, guides, helpers, and loved ones in spirit at any time, we have been taught to distrust the unseen. In doing so, we dim our lights and detach from our true selves.

An intuitive coach and psychic medium can guide us to build that bridge for ourselves once again, to fulfill the purpose of our human experience and allow us to live fully vibrant, meaningful and soul-centered lives. As Lao Tzu said, "When I let go of what I am, I become what I might be."

CHAPTER

Thirteen

God Hear My Call
By Kim Balzan

KIM BALZAN

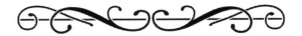

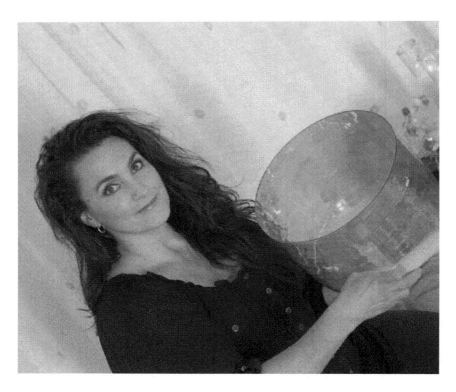

Kim is a holistic practitioner certified in many different modalities, with the most passion going into vibrational sound, working with her alchemy crystal bowls and gongs. She is a Certified Advanced Amrit Method Yoga Nidra Facilitator, Reiki Master Teacher, certified holistic health coach, certified hypnotherapist, and a 200-hour ERYT Kundalini Yoga Teacher, currently finishing Level 2. Her sound studio is located in Scottsdale, Arizona, and she can be reached at 602-577-9408 (mobile), and at kimbalzansound@gmail.com.

Acknowledgments

Thank you to my wonderful, supportive husband and my three beautiful children, and to all of the amazing teachers out in the world who are pushing every day to make a difference.

God Hear My Call
By Kim Balzan

"God, hear my call." That is what I heard on March 19th at 5:55 a.m. many years ago. It was so clear, like a whisper from God or an angel, from something higher than myself. When I had gone to bed the night before, I felt at the lowest point in my life mentally and emotionally. I had a great life—if you were to look at my family, my home, I even had the dog! Inside I felt like I was done, like I had nothing to offer anyone. Nothing brought me happiness. You can have the world, but if the mind is off, nothing matters at all.

This was the day that I would start my journey of self-healing. I knew there was a bigger plan for my life. I started seeking out any modality that I was drawn to—holistic nutrition, hypnotherapy, Reiki, meditation, Yoga Nidra, Kundalini Yoga, and sound—with the belief that there was a reason and a great possibility that it could work. Each of us handles the struggle differently. It doesn't matter how big or small, it feels huge. It's our "stuff," our personal spiritual journey. Others may think, "How could that little thing be such an issue in your life?" We are all unique and one of a kind.

When we start to take time out for ourselves, even if it's five minutes, to begin to be present in the moment and be mindful, change starts. Fear and panic stop when we pause and consciously breathe. Kundalini Yoga, as taught by Yogi Bhajan, changed my life in an instant. Breathwork strengthens our life force and releases toxins from your body and mind. We start to think clearly, and we start to sense a spiritual connection. We feel peace from within, a more positive energy, like we can take on whatever comes at us.

I started off as a professional makeup artist in the television and media industry for over 20 years. The money was amazing; it felt cool and creative, and it was quite different from an average nine-to-five job. I was working in Los Angeles, New York, and eventually Phoenix, where I settled and made my home. After taking a break when my husband and I started our family, I felt there had to be something more out there for me, something bigger to bring me peace and connection. I felt I wanted to work on what's inside instead of what's presented on the outside. I wanted to feel passionate about my life and what I do—to make a difference in the world. That's when Yoga Nidra and Kundalini Yoga fell into my lap and changed my life overnight. Sound completely changed and transformed my life in every way!

Now, I work with private clients and large groups, utilizing these tools of transformation throughout the country to help others awaken and see their true connection to themselves. I am a holistic practitioner, certified in a number of different modalities, with the most passion going into vibrational sound. I work with various sound tools, including gongs, drums, chimes, and a harp, to name a few. My specialty is creating sound experiences, or sound baths, in a gentle way, incorporating breathwork and meditation. I work with a certain type of sound bowl, an alchemy crystal singing bowl made by Crystal Tones, which are the only bowls I use, as they are of the highest quality and have the smoothest sound. They are made with gemstones, minerals, rare crystals, and precious metals. I am also a distributor, and have a lot of alchemy crystal sound bowls in my sound studio to choose from, if you wanted to bring sound in a bigger way into your life. I also facilitate private sound training and mentoring.

What I do each day is my greatest passion. I have seen miracles happen while working with sound and meditation. I personally struggled with fear for a long time—fear of the unknown and fear of what people would think. Something inside me knew that this is what I was meant to do. Working with these tools of transformation is like turning on a light switch. It's that quick, seeing a profound shift or change in someone. My advice is to follow your heart and your gut. You know what your burning desires are. Be fearless, even if you take baby steps. You must take action. You must keep moving toward what you want to do. Keep at it every day. In time, you'll be amazed to see what you have accomplished.

Growing up, I had a huge tree in my front yard that I would sit in for hours. This was my safe place; I felt I was above everything perched up in the air. I have always loved visualization and manifesting what I wanted. I thought it was fun. As a child, I was shy, but I did things that made me feel good, such as art, music, and my great love, cooking. I have always been driven, even at a young age. The hardest part of growing up was losing my father at a young age to a violent crime. I was 16 years old and was forced to grow up overnight. To this day, I honestly have blocks of many years that I have no recollection of. I thought that would be the worst and only tragedy in my life—what could possibly be worse than that event? Then, as an adult and a mother with three children, I lost my 16-year-old nephew to Neuroblastoma cancer. This was a huge blow to my life and my family. After this event, I wasn't sure how to pull myself back up.

What I do today saved my life in every way, and to this day, I am so grateful for the tools that I have found—or maybe they found me. We will always have waves of negative emotions that show up; we will never be happy forever, or sad forever. Life is always changing; it's learning tools to deal with the waves, and knowing that tomorrow is another day. My life is certainly not perfect, but it's pretty great. I still feel fear at times, but I get through it. Life is work; to feel good we need to move and breathe and be conscious of what we are doing each day. We can't run on autopilot.

With all the social media and so much going on out there in the world, it is easy to start comparing ourselves to everyone and everything, thinking we are not up to par. Another struggle of mine has been body image, for probably 90% of my life, but that also stemmed from foods such as the sugary junk I was secretly putting in my body, and that was totally screwing with my mind.

I am so passionate to work with clients and show them all these different alternative modalities, how they affect and impact our lives, and that leading a healthy, productive life is possible.

I have been working with a lot of doctors and cancer centers throughout Arizona. Not only work with sound, but I have also been giving holistic cooking classes to show people how easy it can be to incorporate healthy food into our daily routines.

When I first meet with a client, I ask several questions. Some of the questions I ask are, what do you eat every day? How is your sleep? What kind of music do you listen to? Do you watch TV, what do you watch on TV, and for how long? Some of the most important answers I need to know are what are they eating, and if they are getting enough sleep. What we eat can dictate how our bodies and minds feel, and can be the cause or root of inflammation.

Because I struggled with a sugar addiction from a young age, I feel that I am able to pick up on issues that could completely stem from food. I find that when we make simple changes in our diet, major shifts start to happen. We start to think clearly and experience a reduction in anxiety. You have more energy, and depression starts to lift—simply by changing what we eat.

After a brief consultation, we begin the energy sound session. Sometimes, I will begin with some breathwork to start moving energy. One of the techniques I may use is as follows:

- Either sitting or lying down, begin to focus on the belly

- Close the eyes and begin filling the belly like a balloon

- Hold the breath for at least six seconds.

- Release the breath for the same count

- Hold it for six seconds

Repeat that sequence for up to two minutes. Two minutes may not seem long, but it is when you are consciously breathing.

Other times, I'll use tension and relaxation techniques, which can be done as follows:

- Start with the feet—flex the feet and flex the toes back tight

- Tighten the legs, thighs, and glutes, and hold

- Release

- Pull the navel center back tight and hold, then release

- Make fists with your hands, and tense your arms, so tight that they start to lift off the floor.

Then I will take you through a series of guided visualizations to start relaxing all of your muscles. At this point, I will start playing the sound bowls creating an atmosphere of complete relaxation. The great psychic Edgar Cayce predicted, "Sound will be the medicine of the future."

Continuing with the sound, I incorporate the use of binaural beats through sound bowls, which works on the brain. Some of the benefits of binaural beats are:

- Increased relaxation and deeper meditation

- Increased focus and confidence

- Reduced anxiety, uplift, and reduced depression

When I am finishing up a session and bringing the person out of the experience, most are completely blown away at how deeply they went into a state of meditation. Some tell me about colors they saw or visions of themselves so peaceful. People have said they didn't want to come out of where they were. Their skin tone will look brighter, their eyes will look more alive, and their body will feel relaxed, but energized. Sound brings us there—deep to who we truly are.

I have also experienced that sound can bring back memories that I don't remember ever happening, and clients have also shared this with me. It's fascinating and so rewarding.

Sound can reset our nervous system and help to boost our immune function and decrease inflammation. Dr. Mitchell L. Gaynor was an oncologist who brought sound into his practice, sharing with cancer patients to help soothe them and, he believed, helped heal them. "There's no organ system in the body that's not affected by sound and vibration. You can look at disease as a form of disharmony." ~ Mitchell Gaynor, a pioneer in sound.

Sound and vibration work on the body as a whole. It goes though the bone and bone marrow. It works on the brain and the nervous system, bringing us to a state of well-being and balance. I look at sound vibration almost as if it is a missile that goes right to the spots in the body that are out of balance, or possibly where there was an injury at one time. The sound will find it.

Sound has been around for thousands of years, through instruments such as drums, rattles, chimes, bells and sound bowls, or through voice. Our voice is the most healing tool we have. Sing, hum, chant or whistle, and the vocal toning will help to harmonize and balance your cells. Your vocal cords and the muscles in the back of your throat are all connected to the vagus nerve, which starts at the base of the brain and is the longest nerve in the body. This nerve has a huge effect on our psychological and emotional state.

I believe that in the next five to ten years, sound is going to be mainstream. I am working with cancer centers, with doctors and trauma centers, and in the corporate world. There is so much science to back the modality of sound. People want to feel good, and I find it amazing that people are going back to using some of the oldest modalities on this planet because they work.

We have everything in our bodies to heal, and we need to learn how to use what we have. It all happens through our spiritual journeys. I feel so blessed to do what I do. I treat the body, mind, and spirit as a whole.

There are other, free, resources we can use when we are feeling out of balance. Nature and everything else in the universe are made up of energy. Walk barefoot in the grass. This is extremely grounding and relaxing—connecting to the earth, the animals, the ocean, the sun. Sit with who you are.

CHAPTER

Fourteen

Elderberries: Not Just For Wines And Wands
By Luann Morris Morton

LUANN MORRIS MORTON

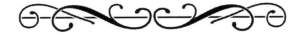

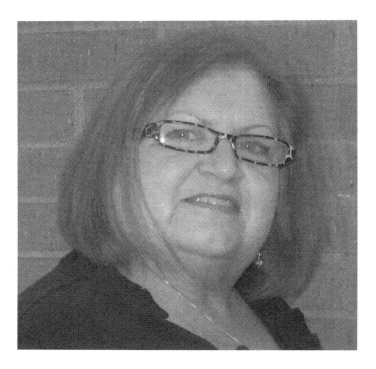

Luann Morris Morton is an herbalist, Licensed Vocational Nurse, Certified Surgical Technologist, Biologist, ordained minister, published author, Reiki Practitioner and professional intuitive card reader. She happily assists individuals to find natural herbal solutions for acute or chronic health issues. Her passion is to help people enjoy healthier lives through nutrition, alternative medications, and herbs. Plants have been a part of her life since she was a small child when she began enjoying the family garden. She retired from corporate life in August 2018 and began her new adventure, Herbal Lu. You can reach Luann at her website: https://herbal-lu1105.vistaprintdigital.com, by phone: 972-664-4342, or by email: herballu1105@gmail.com.

Acknowledgments

A special thank you to my husband, Bill Morton, for his loving support and encouragement. To my sons, John and Robert, and grandson, Luke, thank you. To the Tribe, thank you for having my back in all things: Eleanor Rhodes, Elizabeth Harbin, and Jenny Cabaniss. Thank you to As You Wish Publishing, Kyra and Todd Schaefer, for making this book happen and believing in the authors.

Elderberries: Not Just For Wines and Wands
By Luann Morris Morton

Herbalists, also sometimes called herbal practitioners, are specially trained in the field of herbal medicine. An herbalist uses plants and other natural substances to improve health, promote healing, and deal with symptoms of illness. What is herbal medicine? According to the Journal of Phytomedicine, it is the study of the botany and use of medicinal plants. A medicinal plant is a plant that is used to maintain health. Herbs generally refer to the leafy green or flower parts of a plant, while spices are usually dried and produced from other parts of the plants, including seeds, bark, roots, and fruit. However, in herbal medicine, you will see all parts of the plant referred to as herbs. Herbals are prepared in various different ways. Decoction involves crushing and then boiling the plant material in water to produce a liquid extract. Alcohol extraction involves soaking the plant material in distilled spirits to form a tincture. Infusions happen in my kitchen daily with the preparation of my favorite tea. The active portions of the herbs are coaxed out when hot water is applied to the plant materials and allowed to steep. Syrups are created to make the constituents, extracted from plants through these methods, palatable.

Slowly, with extensive research, I have developed syrups, balms, and combinations of essential oils that family and friends have grown to love. My elderberry syrup was a huge success way before the first processed elderberry items started appearing in the news media. The journey with elderberry began in a search on how to eliminate a chronic cough. My dear friend, Eleanor, was suffering from a 45-year chronic cough due to chronic obstructive pulmonary disease (COPD). Her extensive list of medications triggered my search for something natural that would not interact or counteract her current medications. My scientific research skills took over, and this is what I discovered about the Queen of Herbs, *elderberry*.

Constituents of Elderberry

Elderberries seem to be full of miracle ingredients. According to the USDA National Nutrient Database, elderberries are packed with nutrients, including minerals like iron, potassium, phosphorus, and copper, as well as vitamins A, B, and C, proteins, and dietary fiber. Add in the beneficial organic compounds that function as anti-inflammatory and antioxidant agents in the body, and you have one powerful berry! The syrup also acts as an expectorant and clears out phlegm that can trap foreign agents in your lungs. Elderberry juice is even recommended for people with asthma. Elderberries contain organic pigments, tannins, amino acids, carotenoids, mucilage, sugar, rutin, viburnic acid, and flavonoids. One flavonoid, quercetin, is believed to account for the therapeutic actions of the elderberry flowers and berries. According to test-tube studies, the flavonoids that contain anthocyanins, pigments that give red, purple, and blue plants their rich coloring, are powerful antioxidants, anti-viral, and protect cells against damage.

Many people consider the elderberry plant one of the most powerful for preventing and managing colds and influenza and swear by its antiviral properties. According to a study in the Journal of International Medical Research, flu patients who were given a dosage of elderberry syrup recovered 3-4 days earlier than those who were not given this supplement. Elderberry juice was used to combat a flu epidemic in Panama in 1995. In a randomized, double-blind, placebo-controlled study in Norway, researchers gave either a placebo syrup or elderberry syrup. Patients in the elderberry group reported having flu-like symptoms for less than 48 hours. They also took less over-the-counter medications for the relief of their symptoms. In contrast, Tamiflu took four-and-a-half to five days in a separate study by the World Health Organization, and it is more expensive.

Plant Description

The elder tree is a deciduous shrub or small tree that can grow to 20 feet tall. The leaves are arranged in opposite pairs approximately 3 to 10 inches long. The pairs are arranged on each side of a common stalk with five to seven leaflets with serrated margins. Young stems are hollow. Many species of elderberry (*Sambucus spp.*) are toxic. The branches, leaves, and twigs of all species contain trace elements of cyanide, which can build up in your body and eventually kill you! The elderflowers have both male and female parts which allow you to have berries without having 2 different shrubs. This is called self-pollination. Elderflowers are creamy-white, one-eighth to one-quarter inches in diameter with five petals. Flowering occurs in late spring. The flowers, fresh or dried, can be used to make tea. Elderflowers are known as being beneficial to the respiratory system. Hot elder tea aids the clearing of the lungs. The fruit is a glossy, dark purple to black berry approximately the same diameter as the flowers, produced in drooping clusters in late autumn.

- Some of the benefits of elderberries and elderflowers are:
- Eliminates constipation and boosts the gastrointestinal system
- Beneficial in reducing blood pressure and managing diabetes
- Alleviates respiratory conditions such as cold and cough
- Promotes bone strength and development of new bone tissue
- Aids in eliminating excess cholesterol from the body
- Can be used as a salve for burns, skin irritations, or rashes
- Exhibits preventive properties against some cancers
- Induces wound healing

Cautions when using elderberries and elderflowers:

- Upset stomach
- Diarrhea
- Allergic reactions are possible
- If you are pregnant or breastfeeding first consult your doctor
- Young children should take with caution
- Syrups containing honey should not be consumed by children under 1 year of age.
- If you have a complex liver or kidney disease, consult your doctor.

- If you are taking medications that decrease the immune system, the effectiveness of these medications may be decreased by taking elderberry

A Brief History

Plants have been the basis for medical treatments through much of human history. Elder has often been described as the medicine chest of the country people, and a lot of its medicinal uses are still widely employed by modern herbalists. The "Father of Medicine," Hippocrates, recognized elders' gifts as early as 400 AD. There are recipes for elderberry-based medications dating as far back as ancient Egypt. Elderberry tincture was found in numerous burial tombs. Ancient Egyptians used a salve with elderflowers for their complexion and to heal burns. In 1644, a book dedicated entirely to the virtues of Elder was translated from Latin into English. The author sings the praises of the elder tree in no less than 230 pages. The booklet became so popular that it ran through several editions in both the English and the Latin version. All parts of the plant were mentioned as medicinally useful. The word "elder" is derived from "ellar" or "kindler." The young branches formed tubes that were used as pipes for kindling fires. The botanical name for the elder, *Sambucus,* is from the Greek word *Sambuca*, which means wind instrument. The Romans and the Greeks had a beloved panpipe they called the *Sambuke*, which was also made from young branches. Some Native American tribes also used elderberry branches to make flutes, and they sometimes called the elder "the tree of music." The archaeologist Paul Schumacher reported that he always found elderberries growing near ancient Native American settlements and gravesites. This is not surprising or coincidental. Native Americans found the elderberry plant – the flowers, berries, leaves, bark, and wood – useful in numerous ways, such as poultices, coughs, and skincare.

Elder Folklore

Enchanted folklore surrounds this shrub, and it has long been considered a sacred and strangely magical plant. Elder was said to have powers so amazing it could protect a dwelling from storms, witches, and goblins. It was also said that one could be gifted the power of seeing the future and allowed a glimpse of the faeries if you slept under the elder tree. The fairy tale by Hans Christian Anderson, "Little Elder Tree Mother," is the tale of a little boy who has caught cold and is healed by the elder mother, who comes out of the pot of elder tea. It is a great example of the esteem and respect that was once bestowed upon the elder. According to Danish folklore, there is a female elf in the elder tree who departs at midnight, strolls among the land and fields, and returns before morning.

Similar stories in other European folklore suggest that elder is an enchanted tree, perhaps a true portal to the faerie realm or an embodiment of a crone witch whom you must respect when harvesting from her, so that she won't haunt you for the rest of your days. In astrology, elder is considered a feminine tree and is governed by Venus. Her element is water. Each story told in folklore speaks to powerful magic, but could be modernly defined as the need for humans to acknowledge the plant's power and potent healing abilities.

Personal Experiences

My friends and family will attest to the power of the elderberry. Eleanor swore by the berry that kept her from coughing all night and never wanted to be without it. Since family and friends have been using my elderberry syrup, they have found that not only will it squelch a cough or sore throat, it helps relieve that "I'm getting sick" feeling. Jenny uses it to chase away the feeling that a cold or upper respiratory event is about to take place. She took a tablespoon in the morning for 4 days and never got sick. Elizabeth is happy to take a cough syrup that doesn't cause her to gag or hold her breath. She never hesitates to use my syrup when the cough starts. There is no alcohol in my syrup, only the active ingredients that come with the elderberries and honey to help it go down. I only use sustainable *Sambuca nigra* from reliable sources that guarantee organic, non-GMO, and pesticide-free herbs.

Education

Making medicines for yourself should be done with caution. All ingredients must be purchased through a trusted source. Never wildcraft your herbs unless you have been trained to do so. To be the best herbalist you can be, attend an herbal school to further your education. There are numerous herbal schools to choose from, with different curriculums and emphases, from scientific/evidence-based to the more folk/traditional. Some are online programs, and others are on-site with physical classrooms and classmates. Research different schools and programs and choose one that fits best with your needs and interests.

I chose the East West School of Planetary Herbology. This program is an online self-paced program by Michael and Lesley Tierra. Teachers of teachers, founders of the American Herbalist Guild, and educating for 39 years, they offer over 80 years of combined clinical herbal experience with greater than 10,000 students worldwide. Many of today's well-known practicing herbalists trained at East West, such as Rosalee de la Foret, Roy Upton, and Susan Kramer. All books, curriculum guides, and web access are included with your tuition. You also have unlimited access to online classrooms guided by instructors. To be a clinical herbalist, you must complete a rigorous schedule that will take approximately three years.

Herbals vs. Prescriptions

Herbal medicines are becoming increasingly popular with western cultures as prescription medications and doctor visits become more expensive. Herbs have been used as the basis of Traditional Chinese Medicine, Ayurvedic medicine in India, and modern medicine. Modern pharmaceuticals have their origins in herbal medicines, and some drugs are still extracted as compounds from raw herbs, such as aspirin (from the willow tree), digitalis (foxglove), atropine (nightshade), codeine (poppy), morphine (poppy), scopolamine (jimsonweed) and quinine (cinchona tree). Approximately 25 percent of modern drugs used in the United States have been derived from plants. The World Health Organization estimates that 80 percent of the population of some Asian and African countries presently use herbal medicine for some aspect of primary health care. The percentages in the United States are also on the rise as the public has become more educated on herbal medicines and the cost of health care and prescription medicines escalate.

Are you ready to try an herbal? Purchase ingredients from any reputable brick and mortar or online store. There are lots of recipes. This is one example for making elderflower tea. Many swear that this tea chases away their cold symptoms.

Gather the following ingredients:

- Elderflowers, dried or fresh
- Filtered spring water
- Honey, local is the best

Step 1. Measure 3 ½ cups of water, bring to a boil.

Step 2. Fill a 1-quart jar with elderflowers to the shoulder of the jar.

Step 3. Cover plant material with the boiled water. Stir.

Step 4. Steep plant material in hot water covered for 30 minutes. Strain well.

Step 5. Add honey to desired sweetness. Drink warm or cold to your preference.

From small beginnings, I have grown into an herbalist. Plants have been in my life since I was a small child attending the family garden. It gives me joy and satisfaction to work with herbal remedies. I am currently working on a cough drop using the elderberry decoction that will be portable and more practical. Soon, I will begin work on a throat lozenge with slippery elm that will aid in soothing a scratchy throat and will be a lifesaver for people who are speakers, singers, or teachers. I have also developed a hand balm for a friend that teaches Crystal Reiki healing and chakra alignment. This balm softens at the warm touch of your fingers and coats your hands with shea butter and essential oils to enhance your healing energy. Another future endeavor will be roll-on essential oils to deal with emotional feelings such as stress, anxiety, and insomnia.

Wines and Wands

Other than medicinal purposes, the elderberry has a long history of use for food and drink. Elderberry pie, jam and jelly, tarts, flavored drinks, and of course wine are a few of its better-known uses. Sometimes referred to as the "Englishman's grape," the common elderberry has been used to make wine for hundreds—possibly thousands—of years. If you have no desire to make medicinal preparations, wine would be a fun step to take. The elder tree even took a trip to Hogwarts. As authors are known to do with everyday objects, J.K. Rowling added to the elder tree lore: "Did you know that the most powerful wand in the Wizarding World of Harry Potter is made of *Sambucus* wood and is known as the Elder Wand?" It is safe to say; the life of the elder tree is and will always be revered far and wide. It encompasses many uses and traditions that are not likely to be replaced any time soon.

CHAPTER

Fifteen

Reiki: The Power In Your Palms
By Megan Moffitt

MEGAN MOFFITT

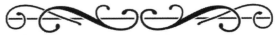

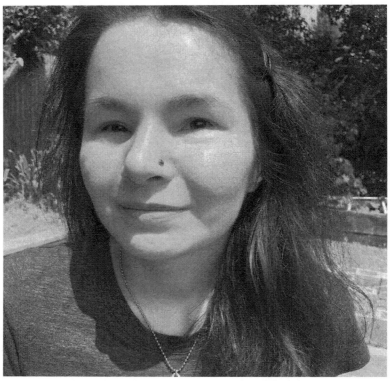

Megan Moffitt is a Reiki Master who works with women to help them relax and release stress to improve their overall well-being. Her mission is to be of service to others through the use of her gifts of compassion and empathy, and to make a positive difference in the world. You can reach Megan online at facebook.com/1lovereiki.

Acknowledgments

Thank you to Anne, my wonderful friend and teacher, who inspired me to discover gifts I didn't know I had. Thank you to my mother, Sherrie, for everything since day one. You were the one to show me what working hard to achieve your dreams looks like. Thank you for supporting mine.

Reiki: The Power In Your Palms
By Megan Moffitt

All my life, I have been plagued by near-debilitating migraines. During my childhood and teenage years, they occurred with such frequency and severity that I often had to stay home from school or leave early, unable to stand the agonizing pain accompanied by nausea and vomiting. I had been diagnosed with multiple brain aneurysms as a little girl, and, as sudden, intense headaches are one of the common signs of a ruptured aneurysm, there were also a handful of trips to the emergency room while I was growing up. My doctors, concerned about weakening these already-compromised blood vessels and causing a potentially fatal brain bleed, advised me not to take over-the-counter NSAIDs like aspirin and ibuprofen to treat my migraines. Instead, I relied upon a prescription-strength analgesic to get me through the most excruciating episodes.

Unfortunately, the prescribed drugs seemed to become less and less effective over time. I remember putting ice packs and cool cloths on my forehead in an attempt to soothe the horrible throbbing in my skull. Sometimes my mother would lie on my bed next to me and massage my head. I heard somewhere that caffeine was supposed to be beneficial in combatting headaches, so occasionally when I had to leave school in the middle of the day, I would ask to stop for coffee on the way home. But usually, I wanted to sleep through the agony if I could. After years of suffering, I began to think there was nothing I could do to make the pain go away.

Then, when I was about sixteen, an English assignment unexpectedly led me to discover a new way of dealing with my migraines. The assignment was to interview someone about their life, then use that information to write a creative nonfiction story about them. I chose to interview a classroom aid named Anne, and one of the things she told me was that she was a Reiki Master. I had never heard of Reiki before, let alone a Reiki Master, but I was instantly intrigued by Anne's description of a Japanese form of energy work that encourages relaxation and stress relief. She also showed me a simple technique for using it on myself.

The next time I had a headache, I remembered what Anne had taught me, and was both surprised and amazed when my pain disappeared. Was this a coincidence, a one-time event, or true hope for relief? Determined to find out more, I dove into an online search.

I quickly learned that Reiki is based on the principle that life force energy flows through a series of seven points called *chakras*, aligned along the length of the spinal column. If the chakras become blocked or imbalanced, it can contribute to physical, mental, emotional, and/or spiritual health issues. A practitioner gently places their hands on a client's chakra points and uses the power of intention to send positive energy through their palms into the body, thereby helping it enter a relaxed state from which it can begin to heal. A Reiki Master is one who has received three levels of training and attunements that enable him or her to train other practitioners. I also learned that Reiki has been found to be so effective in improving overall well-being that many hospitals and medical facilities across the country now offer it to their patients as a supplemental treatment option.

Over the next seven years, I continued to pursue my knowledge of Reiki with passion and a deep sense of soul purpose that I didn't fully understand. I remembered something that my grandmother had told me when I was perhaps five or six—we are put here to help others. Reiki, more than anything else in my life, felt like the way I was being called to help, so although I didn't truly know what I was doing, I kept doing it.

Finally, in 2013, I completed all three levels of Reiki training and received the Master attunement, a sort of right-of-passage ceremony that's intended to boost a person's innate energetic gifts. Words cannot adequately express what it meant to me to have accomplished my dream after so long. Yet, in truth, it was still only the beginning of my journey. To this day, I am constantly learning, and each lesson makes me a better human being. Reiki teaches me every day to be grateful, compassionate, and empathetic. It reminds me to have confidence in myself and to trust my intuition. It opens doors to new opportunities, such as partnering with Anne, who first set me on this path, to teach Reiki, participating in community Reiki circles, working at healing arts fairs, and building friendships with other practitioners. Last but certainly not least, it brings peace and joy to my heart.

If you're a newcomer to Reiki, you might be wondering how someone can use this holistic modality if they've been given little or no proper instruction. And if training isn't necessary—as it wasn't for me in reducing the pain from my migraines—why bother with it at all? What would be the benefit of receiving a treatment from a practitioner as opposed to treating oneself?

Many people who have studied Reiki have been taught that it must remain a closely guarded secret, never to be discussed with anyone who has not also been trained. This notion has persisted throughout the decades since the late 1930s when Reiki was first introduced in the Western world. At that time, there were few Reiki Masters, the most well-known of them being a woman named Hawayo Takata. Mrs. Takata strictly forbade her students to take notes of any kind and discouraged them from altering or deviating from the methods she imparted to them, saying if they did they would no longer truly be practicing Reiki.

Interestingly, it was this lack of written records—and, therefore, no materials for new Masters to refer back to—that virtually guaranteed Reiki would grow and evolve. Today, an ever-increasing number of practitioners are of the opinion that, unlike certain other types of energy work, Reiki can be done by anyone, whether they have had any formal training or not. Reiki relies on intention and intuition more than anything else, which means that we all already have within ourselves the power and ability to be healers. You don't need anyone else's permission, or any special tools or knowledge. You must simply learn to follow your heart.

That said, while giving yourself Reiki may seem like the quicker, easier option, it's not always the most advantageous one. Because you are the one doing the work, you might not be able to fully disengage and be at rest. As the client, you do nothing beyond removing your shoes and making yourself comfortable in a face-up position on a massage table. A good practitioner will tailor the session to your needs and preferences by offering pillows or blankets, making adjustments to lighting, playing soothing music, using crystals to enhance energies, adding aromatherapy, and so on.

During the treatment, the practitioner will also systematically assess the movement of energy through all of your chakras. Training will have taught them a basic awareness of the biological systems and psychological, emotional, and spiritual conditions that correspond to each one. Experience will have taught them to recognize what blocked energy feels like, and they will intuitively understand how to help release it. At the end of the session, they will take time to discuss with you what they observed and answer any questions. If, for example, they found your sacral chakra to be imbalanced, and you're curious as to what that means, the knowledge they have acquired through the combination of study and practice will allow them to offer some ideas. As Reiki practitioners are neither therapists nor medical professionals, they cannot make diagnoses or prescribe medication. Instead, their responsibility is to explain to you the physical and nonphysical functions of the sacral so that you can reflect upon what might be causing the imbalance and decide how you would like to proceed with addressing it.

Reiki training also involves teaching students to respect their clients' personal space, and to be mindful of boundaries and potential triggers. Some people suffer from pain and/or anxiety as a result of experiencing trauma and may not wish to be touched directly. Therefore it is important for the practitioner to explain to the client beforehand that Reiki usually involves light touch, but if that is not desirable, the treatment can be done by simply holding the hands above the chakras. Should a client express feelings of discomfort at any point, the practitioner must communicate with him or her to determine what they can do to remedy the problem or, if the client wishes, end the session immediately.

This is merely the proverbial tip of the iceberg with regard to what you can learn from a legitimate Reiki teacher. Some things won't necessarily be applicable if you're only intending to self-treat, but it's useful to be aware of them anyway, and absolutely essential if you ever choose to give Reiki to others. Even if you never practice on anyone else, it's wise to remember these lessons when receiving Reiki from another. An untrained practitioner is not likely to know that certain etiquette is to be followed or be able to provide vital feedback, which could lead to an unsatisfactory experience. Remember, even Reiki practitioners seek treatment from other professionals from time to time. Though they could and possibly do work on themselves, they understand that being the client allows one to relax more fully and, therefore, reap greater benefits.

That said, knowing how to give yourself a treatment is extremely valuable. Maybe you have a busy schedule and find it difficult to make time for a Reiki appointment. If you know where the chakras are located within your body and how to position your hands atop them, you can give yourself five-minute treatments while lying in bed in the morning or right before you go to sleep at night. This will help keep your energy up and in balance until you are next able to visit your practitioner for a full session.

Cost is another factor to consider. The price of a Reiki treatment can vary depending on where you live, and if regular sessions aren't in the budget knowing how to treat yourself in between will help you prolong the healing benefits and stay in balance.

Then, of course, there are those times when you need Reiki now and can't wait for a practitioner. Maybe you had a long, stressful day and desperately need to relax. Maybe you have a severe headache, and nothing else is helping. Maybe it's three a.m., and you can't sleep. Self-treatment to the rescue! Remember that while Reiki is a powerful healing tool, it is meant to be used in concurrence with your conventional medical care or treatment regimen. If you have an emergency or are concerned about something, seek immediate medical attention.

If you are interested in self-treating with Reiki, here is a simple exercise to help you get started. It consists of seven affirmations, one for each chakra. These affirmations are meant to teach you the names of the chakras, as well as their functions. Directions are given to help you locate each chakra and to instruct you on hand positions. Place your hands gently over each point, speak the corresponding affirmation out loud, rest in that position for as long as feels necessary, then move to the next one. The first step is to find a quiet, comfortable place to sit or lie down where you will not be interrupted or distracted.

Chakra Affirmations Exercise

Root: Located at the base of the spine. Lightly place your hands just above your pubic bone and say, "Today, I am strength. I hold my power in my root chakra. I meet adversity with courage and resilience."

Sacral: Located approximately two inches below the navel. Lightly place your hands below your navel and say, "Today, I am compassion. I hold my power in my sacral chakra. I treat myself and everyone around me with loving kindness."

Solar plexus: Located approximately two inches above the navel. Lightly place your hands above your navel and say, "Today, I am confidence. I hold my power in my solar plexus chakra. I accomplish everything I set my mind to with grace and ease."

Heart: Located in the center of the chest. Lightly place your hands over your heart and say, "Today, I am faith. I hold my power in my heart chakra. I trust in all that is good and of the light."

Throat: Located at the base of the throat. Lightly place your hands on your throat and say, "Today, I am truth. I hold my power in my throat chakra. I speak my thoughts with honesty and clarity."

Third Eye: Located in the center of the forehead between the eyebrows. Lightly place your hands on your forehead and say, "Today, I am intuition. I hold my power in my third eye chakra. I hear the wisdom of my inner voice and allow it to guide me in the right direction."

Crown: Located at the top of the head. Lightly place your hands on top of your head and say, "Today, I am gratitude. I hold my power in my crown chakra. I give thanks for all that I have been blessed with in this life."

Reiki has the potential to positively affect one's life in countless ways. Indeed, what began as a remedy for my migraines has become an integral part of my life. Similar to prayer, Reiki is fueled by intention, so it is easily applied to any situation for which a specific outcome is desired, such as sending Reiki to aid in the recovery of a sick pet, to console an upset child, or to keep yourself safe while traveling. It is one of the most versatile holistic modalities, and is equally accessible to everyone, whether they want to give or receive. If, like me, you feel a calling to learn and share Reiki, don't hesitate or doubt yourself. You were born with the power to do beautiful and meaningful things, and once you embrace that power, your life, and the world around you, will begin to shift.

CHAPTER

Sixteen

Working With Prosperity
By Melissa Kim Corter

MELISSA KIM CORTER

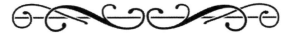

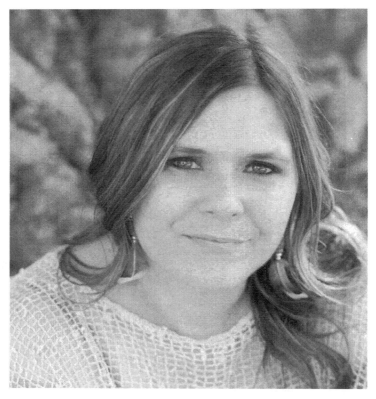

Melissa Kim Corter is a certified hypnotherapist, shamanic practitioner, and intuitive advisor, mentoring creatives, healers, and business owners to create and receive success. She's certified in over 35 healing modalities, and has a unique ability to sense energy blockages and self-defeating patterns cycling through the nervous system and subconscious mind. Through her heightened intuition, Melissa hones in on specific emotions and ages that blockages occurred, providing clarity and tools to release the blockages. Her specialty is clearing emotions sabotaging prosperity and visibility.

Acknowledgments

To my grandmother, you taught me the power of money and all it can do for and to people. I am grateful for the healing I have received, and the gifts my pain created in service to others. Thank you for being one of my greatest teachers, hard lessons in love, life, and money.

Working With Prosperity
By Melissa Kim Corter

Becoming an intuitive healer and certified hypno-therapist was not something I wanted. Funny thing about this universe: we get what we need, not always what we want. The healing arts mysteriously and quietly pulled me in. Because I felt deeply broken, I started to seek various therapies and modalities.

After a little kicking and screaming, tons of resistance, and a helpful mentor, I finally accepted my abilities as an intuitive. I call my higher-self "the all-knowing, wise part of me," and this part was not going to let me hide my gifts from the world. Interestingly enough, the more I tried to deny them, the stronger they became. This caused so much massive discomfort that I needed to find professionals to help me understand my experiences.

My intuition was sharp and incredibly accurate, yet my confidence was almost nonexistent. To handle my in-security, I continued to learn, taking class after class. Today, I hold over 30 certifications; I share this not to brag, but to paint a picture of how deeply I lacked confidence. I believed if I could learn one more thing, I may be valuable and good enough.

Confidence was only the beginning of the emotional obstacles. As I stepped into my work and began to do it professionally, it didn't take long to realize how many others in the healing arts industry were struggling financially— talented people doing good work and serving others with their gifts. So why were they all financially broke and in debt? Lightworkers fighting to keep their lights turned on, healers breaking down with adrenal fatigue, caught in competition and acting out of integrity to get the sale. It was starting to become disheartening to me, and I did not think I would survive financially or emotionally doing this work.

I was shocked to discover amazing people who were helping people heal, releasing trauma, shifting generational patterns, and at the same time, they were not running profitable businesses. They were barely keeping their heads above water, many working a "real" job while they did their healing work as a side hustle. This pattern cycled all around me, and rarely did I encounter someone in the field living an abundant and prosperous life.

I witnessed transformational healing, past life re-gressions, and magnificent psychic mediums, only to also watch these same people put out a sad looking paper cup to retrieve any bit of financial compensation someone might give them. They were underpaid while continuing to over serve. Fear began to surface as it brought the lens to my life and situation, for I, too, was not letting myself receive for the work.

It was a challenge finding a rhythm to supporting myself as a massage therapist, hypnotherapist, and intuitive guide. Massage therapy eventually dropped away from my services after I developed my intuitive skills; working with the physical body opened up my intuition to new levels. It served me to hone my craft, and it created a safe space for me to explore the guidance I was receiving as I worked with my clients. Intuitive information dropped into my consciousness in the form of lights all around the client's body as they relaxed on the table, this was the beginning of a whole new world developing for me.

Stepping into the intuitive work, I created another interesting pattern. I began to attract all of those same practitioners and healers who struggled financially. They now wanted my services and were referred due to my style of helping people uncover and break patterns and cycles. To be honest, I was a bit disappointed, as scarcity, fear, and financial struggle were the last topics I wanted to work with.

This began the process of understanding that my internal world was creating an external reflection through these people and their struggles. If it comes to your door, there is something there for you to learn about yourself. Everything in this universe becomes externalized for us to learn and grow from.

As the stubbornness began to melt away, gratitude took over; I was good at helping people see their patterns, and helping them create new healthy ones. For this to take place, I had to recognize the level of lack that also existed within myself. These clients offered me the gift of seeing the unhealed aspects of myself through their struggles and patterns. This opened me up to helping myself and them to shift the paradigm instead of feeling frustrated about it. It assisted me in shifting my stories and patterns of lack.

Working through my relationship to money allowed more of it to come in. In fact, I attracted an unexpected large sum of a few hundred thousand dollars from doing this work. This was a gift, providing the time I needed to focus on my work and continue to develop my business. Everything was going well, until one pivotal moment as I opened my computer to check my bank account. I stared at this number for what felt like an hour; the number was $72,000. For most of us, this number would be appreciated, but I hated it. It didn't feel like enough, and it became symbolic of all of the money I was now letting slip through my hands.

Defeat and complete fear ruled my mind. Not long ago, hundreds of thousands of dollars were in that same account—where had it all gone? It felt like I was hemorrhaging money, every day seeing it dwindle. This moment revealed a life-changing insight, the dollar amount had no bearing on my life, yet I could see my perception of it was dictating how I felt about myself and my value.

The next morning, before my eyes even opened, I woke with panic in my belly, and tension in my head. The anxiety overwhelmed my body and brought thoughts of fear and failure. In the exact moment I was in fear, my higher-self engaged and was speaking to me loud and clear. Until this point in my life, fear had drowned out any sense of knowing, but for whatever reason, this moment was different, and I was aware of both experiences happening together.

My higher-self clearly stated, "Get your journal, keep your eyes slightly closed, and write exactly what you are afraid of right now." I scribbled like a madwoman, some of it illegible, yet I knew something big was happening.

I could feel it, and then as I wrote and wrote, tears began flowing, dripping down onto my page. All of the anxiety I held started to turn into words, and the words were:

You are failing

You cannot do this

It's not working, and you are going to lose it all

Sobbing uncontrollably, I let the words flow through me and out of my pen. More came forth, they became deeper, heavier, and more intense as the pen moved in jagged and sharp motions on the page, ink disappearing as it touched upon tears that dissipated as the droplets touched down on the page.

The magic of the moment then revealed itself, as a warm, calm sensation washed over me, erasing all anxiety from my system. I felt a deep inner stillness while my mind fought, trying to cling to the fearful thoughts I processed through my body. My higher-self guided me to breathe through it, and to rest in the moment of stillness. The guidance continued, with my inner voice stating to "program my nervous system" to recognize this peaceful feeling as my new emotional set point.

The new peace of being was to become a state for me to strive to feel on a regular basis. I was also told, through this stream of consciousness, to regulate my energy and consciously direct my mind and mood, to harmonize my vibrational frequency. I could then begin powerfully attracting my desires with greater ease. Along with the manifestations, it would also help my physical body heal, and rejuvenate because of the parasympathetic response I was creating with my mind and body together as one.

After a few moments of sitting in this peaceful, blissful state, I was amazed at how often my mind kept trying to regain control over the situation; then I had my Eckhart Tolle moment of "Who and what is the mind, who and what is the stillness, and who or what is witnessing them both?" I used my breath to bring me back and to release the residual emotions the mind had begun to generate. After this happened, something else shifted for me, I downloaded an entire prosperity process to work through for the old stuck emotions in my nervous system and limiting beliefs within my subconscious mind.

The process began with writing to release emotions and the dense energy in my body. Then, it shifted to using the breath to connect to my higher-self and the sympathetic state of being. Next, I was guided to write a list of negative thoughts I held about money. Each one led me to a story of my past, a time I left behind a part of my essence and brought forth a negative belief or agreement. I was shown my age, the unexpressed emotion, and the agreement. I then witnessed myself through the eyes of a child seeing the situation in real time. This is where I discovered that the adult me could share a new perspective with the child, to see it differently and from another angle. As soon as the child could recognize this, it brought an immediate shift to her consciousness and allowed the energy to fully integrate into my being.

After the energetic integration occurred, I was guided to use a new affirmation or mantra to help program my nervous system like I did for the peaceful state of being.

This experience was life-changing for me, my business tripled, my clients started opening to receive, and the work helped me begin to discover additional common themes for my clients in why they were not allowing money in or receiving.

This process took years to refine, and everyone I use it with works through it at an individual pace. I recognized each person had a varying degree of being able to rest in the still space; others struggled to breathe and feel the emotion in their body. This could be painful if they have unresolved emotion, which there usually is, and the external situation became the indicator of this inner conflict. I am excited to share a beautiful piece of this process here with you in this chapter. My intention is for you to experience the joy life has to offer and to always know that you are enough. Prosperity flows as we discover our innate value internally, not our external world or material possessions and bank accounts.

Preparing for the process

In the following experience, you can create the same peaceful state I felt when this process came to me. Anyone can do it, and you do not need to be a writer, or have any confidence in your writing at all. In fact, not knowing anything about writing may serve you in detaching from the outcome as you practice. A critical aspect of this exercise is truly letting yourself relax and get lost in it. Learning to let go of control is something many of us struggle with, and yet, it's the exact ingredient necessary to create profound results in this experience. Letting go allows inner spaciousness, providing the mind a break from holding everything together.

The result of this practice can create a profound shift for those who take the time to use it. The mind can be sneaky in trying to convince you to skip the work, which is actually a subtle form of resistance or even self-sabotage.

Do not edit or censor as you write, give yourself permission to write freely and openly. We can unconsciously stop a process as emotion begins to surface by becoming a critic of our words, written or spoken. Instead of editing or trying to change what you write, lean into the feelings and allow them to move through you. Stay present, committed, and conscious to the act of writing and letting go. Do not worry about sentence structure either. This format of writing is geared to help the release of trapped energy within your mind and body.

Prepare with a notebook or journal and writing utensil. Free yourself of distractions, shut off electronic devices, and find a quiet space to be present and comfortable in. You will be writing for five minutes straight, this may seem challenging after the first few minutes. When you "empty" the emotion, energy, and thoughts, the space opens up within you.

Working with the energy of prosperity

There are three steps to the process:

1. Empty the mind with writing
2. Connect to the breath to create inner space and calm
3. Open to your higher-self

Step One: Let's walk through the process together. Grab your pen and paper, as you bring to mind an uncomfortable emotion, preferably one you feel is connected to money. Close your eyes and keep generating this uncomfortable feeling, trusting the process, and letting it come up from within you. Take it to the paper now, writing everything you are feeling and wanting to let go of when it comes to this feeling and money. Continue writing for five minutes (or longer if you are not yet complete) without interruption.

Step Two: This step is all about learning the power of your breath to activate a calming effect on the entire body and system. It puts the mind at ease, which then helps the body rest, digest, and heal. Deepen your breath and let it feel easy as you slow your inhalations and exhalations, taking your time to draw the breath in, and to allow it to flow out. Breathe through your nose to soothe you. After a few moments of breathing intentionally, you may notice you have an individual rhythm, your breath can teach you a lot about how you think and how you process situations in life.

Step Three: This step is to remember your natural state of being. It is the one that gets you into alignment with prosperity consciousness. Close your eyes, and feel this spaciousness within you. Get familiar with deeply feeling through the body. Ask your higher-self, "What can I do to let money in?" then sit, feel, and breathe, and see what floats to the surface. This may take time to practice—if the mind becomes busy, go back to step one or step two.

Additional prompts to ask in step three:

- What do I need to know, do, or work on to improve my relationship with my finances?
- Is there an action I can take to shift my mindset?

As you practice you'll shift your prosperity energy and point of attraction. You have everything you need within—with this belief, all is possible.

CHAPTER

Seventeen

Come Into Balance
By Michele J. Halverson

MICHELE J. HALVERSON

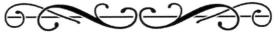

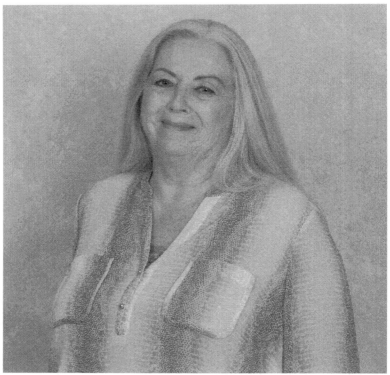

Michele is a hypnotherapist, a Reiki Master, and a distance healer who has studied over a dozen modalities to learn healing from many perspectives. Her passion is sound healing, especially with Solfeggio tuning forks. Her other passion is helping folks deal with death. She spends time with her grandchildren, as this too can be great medicine. You may contact her at ReikiChick111@gmail, and you may text her at 480-234-8119.

Acknowledgments

I am deeply grateful for the help of Karen Balderrama, Oneness facilitators: Rev. Kerry Chinn, Miguel Angel Lopez, Dr. Jim Lane, and Cheryl Cross. Fr. Jorge from The Shrine of Holy Wisdom. Hypnotherapy teacher: Marilyn Gordon. Mike Dooley and his Notes From the Universe. New thought teachers, Abraham-Hicks. Sara O'Meara and The Little Chapel. Yvonne Fedderson: *Miracle Healing: God's Call*. Florence Scovel-Shinn: *The Game of Life and How to Play It*. My children Melissa and Christyne, their children Kenley, Aurie, and Aspen. They have given me more joy than I could possibly imagine.

Come Into Balance
By Michele J. Halverson

Moving much of my young life, I experienced extremes: weather, pollens, toxins, and vaccinations for traveling abroad. A military brat—one of six—seen and not heard, and spankings were the solution to noisy kids. We got chickenpox, measles, and mumps. If we were contagious, doctors made house calls. Today, thank God for the Medical Medium and his books teaching that nutrition is real medicine, why our original maladies are still causing havoc, and what we can do outside of prescriptions.

When my children were graduating (2000), I was free to take classes for myself. I had lived in Silicon Valley and, now, was 90 minutes east. I heard about weekend classes in the Bay Area and budgeted accordingly.

Hypnotherapy classes were eye-opening, transformational, and healing, plus there were like-minded souls. Bonus: we did not have to take a lot of notes, as we were learning to tune into our higher selves for answers. We met practitioners from the Bay Area who specialized in addiction, weight loss, smoking, cancer, and my mouth dropped. I attended classes in other specialties such as color therapy, shamanism, crystal healing, and my all-time favorite, Emotional Freedom Technique (EFT). EFT was continuing to develop. I would travel, even fly, to where Gary Craig was holding a weekend seminar. These programs were evolving—extra healing for all. He said, "Try it on everything." I did. I taught it to strangers and little neighbor kids.

San Francisco offered Shaman classes on Friday nights. I was a student of shamanism for two years. By now our luck had changed, additional money allowed my husband and I both new cars. Michael Harner offered two-day classes in the city. The energy in those large groups was exceptional. This man went around the world to countries that were once forbidden to practice shamanism, and he reintroduced it to them! Now there is a calling. In his presence, we all excelled. May I also mention that we are not in this work alone. We call in our ancestors, and they do the actual work. We hold space, which is the intention, as does the recipient. So, talking to trees, reading rocks, journeying, learning to understand nature, and channeling were coming fast. Drumming was magic. My idea of meditating is with a window open, listening to the trees, the birds, and the messages that come in clearly. If near water, that sound as well. Once, near Sedona, I stayed in an Airbnb that had the sounds of a shamanic event. It turned out to be cicadas (insects) that make some beautiful music. I felt in sync with nature.

In hypnotherapy class, one classmate was a Reiki Master Teacher, and she provided my first attunement. My hands used to get "too hot" to rest on my body in an aerobics class at cooldown time. It happened to be in a church facility where we prayed for folks at the end. Here I realized I could see breast cancer in people. It was always pretty. It diminished when prayed over. So, while not a medical intuitive, I was getting information. The commute and my new car without a passenger allowed me to listen to books on tape or cd. I could hear a book in three days and complete a holistic seminar with numerous speakers in about a week. I was soaking it all up. Reiki was offered online for free as Reiki Secrets from the U.K. I signed up, and within 24 hours, I was in my morning shower and felt the same energy as in my original Reiki One attunement. People at my work would come to me and ask me to touch a spot on them because it hurts. I did not hang a shingle or mention my classes, except to my husband. It did not seem strange to me. When they were in pain, they came to see me on their break.

One day when the stress of my marriage was causing tension across my back, I remembered a Louise Hay book saying, "What you most need is what you most need to give!" So I found a massage school two hours from home in San Jose that had a 100 hour, two weeks and two weekends long class. It cost me a two-week paycheck and gas. I told my boss I needed two weeks off. All good. The bonus: I got two massages a day for two weeks. Hello! And after graduation, my husband got a massage whenever he wanted on my table at home. He bragged at work. Win-win.

Within a year, divorce was proceeding. We had different definitions of love. I was releasing him to find what he believed he needed. I was free. The kids had seen a lot of unpleasantries between us, and I wanted them to know they could have any relationship standards they wanted.

So after becoming a Reiki One practitioner, it took me two years to do Reiki on myself first each day. Two years! But I finally got that I was an instrument which God or my divine could work through. I need to polish that instrument. My issues began to diminish. I gave up wine nightly as it conflicted with my intention. I got my Reiki Two and Three certifications in the Bay Area. I learned there were other types of Reiki besides Usei. You pay, you study, you practice, you get attuned and certified. I took the first one online as a prerequisite to the one with no symbols, La Ho Chi. You can use hand mudras instead of symbols. Fast forward 20 years and you no longer have to tell the energy where to go (emotional, physical, or mental). The world is evolving.

Around Y2K, I was in Ohio at a holistic shop, The Gentle Wind. A flier announced Solfeggio tuning fork training in chakra colors. Before I signed up, I attended a Gift of Light Expo, and the first vendor inside the door was David Hulse and his SomaEnergetics crew. They gave seven-minute tune-ups while we sat on a stool. Six practitioners were tuning folks up. David used a pendulum and showed me each chakra was open. Seven minutes later, I am sitting up straighter, feeling as if a fountain was coming out the top of my head. David again used the pendulum on my chakras, and it spun flat out like a dinner plate instead of the smaller circles before the tune-up. I had brought enough money for one set and took them home with me. I signed up for his Level One practitioner class and took it with my sisters. One said she remembered doing this in an Egyptian lifetime. I do know it worked amazingly well. Another sister who did not buy a set, hurt her knees, and I used my set to reduce her swelling and pain. Another sister who was on her way to becoming a hoarder started giving tune-ups for free to her martial arts teachers. Her life changed. She could have parties at her home because she opened it up. Progress!

These forks do not go out of tune, do not use batteries, nor cords.

Later while traveling across the country, the Level Two Soma practitioner class was happening where I was stopping, which I took as a sign. Level Two practitioner now. By 2006, I was working the San Francisco Whole Life Expo with David Hulse as part of his crew, giving Solfeggio tune-ups to the public. Ten years later, David Hulse and Tim came to Sedona to introduce spa workers to other forks available. Now living in Phoenix, I went, trained, and counted my forks. I own all the forks he sells. Just playing with the forks raises your vibration. You can increase the vibration of your water and food with the MI fork. It is gold and sold separately for this purpose. Imagine if everyone had one. There are love vibe forks, earth, moon, crystal, archangel forks, OM, brain balancing, the planetary group, and more. Body tuners have round weights, so the vibration lasts longer in your body. The others are not too loud, but you must tap them away from the ears, usually to another fork or hockey puck or something similar.

Facebook has at least two groups (Australia and the U.K.) that teach about using tuning forks as prescriptions for causes of pain such as the sinus infections I used to get. Eileen Day McKusick from the U.S. explores the human biofield and gives free—or almost free—work on your biofield through group phone calls or maybe skype or zoom. She has a beauty fork for less than a jar of good face cream. One must use these tools for them to work. So, pardon any remaining wrinkles right now. Where is my fairy god-mother? Laughing her butt off, I am sure.

Traveling monks offered Blue Medicine Buddha training in the same town I lived in about six years ago. Small cost, small sacrifice (fasting) to purify your vessel, short travel, I am in! No big secrets, just trust, set your intention, and do team up with this great being. Green Tara, a few years later, same thing. I was looking for the magic that allowed one to remove pain from others, especially those afraid to die. With permission, of course. I am no one's fairy godmother. Another healer told me to blast that energy to a burn unit at a hospital. Many classes later, one person put it bluntly, "Michele, you have all the answers, go inside and get them." She handed me back my cash, and we went to dinner.

The last guru I took training from was living in Southern California. He said to reach for the highest dimension you can imagine. He said, "Surrender to the higher realms and your person. Like, prostrate yourself at their feet." That was a valuable piece to this puzzle.

There is one additional thing—you cannot fix people who do not want to be fixed. Secondary gain is a term I learned in hypnotherapy. For example, a woman may be large because she can keep from being propositioned. Some folks get a lot of help from the government and other beautiful souls so, should they lose their disability, they would have to go back to working, cooking and cleaning and shopping themselves without these "paid friends." Some folks like to brag that they have been to the best shamans and healers, with no positive results. Well, folks, you have to open that door, to allow healing. It is not enough to pay or ask. You must want it and appreciate it for it to stick. I have enjoyed sound healing of many types and love going to gongs, crystal and Tibetan bowls and much more being orchestrated by one person or two. Drumming circles rock my world. Find what rocks yours.

One of my favorite practices learned as a student of shamanism is what I lovingly refer to as Humpty Dumpty. This is where one will journey with the intent to unburden yourself. You become your power animal or choose one that you resonate with today. I became a crow. Now see yourself enjoying life, then see your death. It is all good. You are in pieces down below. Your soul self looks down to see the parts all separated. Not only the physical, but the ego-self: the greedy self, the needy self, the addicted self. Now the recreation is the best, as you only choose the parts you wish to contain going forward. When you put yourself back together, miraculously you are new and unburdened. To test out your unique self, you find a mirror or, in my case, I flew to the ocean and chose some big rocks that were being splashed with salt water as the tide came in. I felt the salt-water, and it did not sting as it would if I was cut open. I was healed, whole, and fabulous, ready to continue on the earth plane without the negativity. Great makeover. So our condition is temporary. Imagine that. Other cultures do this for their new year. For me, this was almost child-like.

Similarly, The Transformation Game (created by the Findhorn Foundation in Scotland) was mind-blowing to me to find out how we are all gifted at birth. We have to part with some of those gifts to evolve. Spoiler alert! We get upgrades as we let go of others. Four people can play for an hour or two and learn so much. It seems created specifically for us.

Sara O'Meara has The Little Chapel in Paradise Valley, Arizona. People around the world who received healing there, return to testify. Over 45 years ago, Sara had cancer and was expected to live for three more months. At a healing service in Southern California, she was healed and told she was to go on and hold healing services as well. She has a world-wide charity, ChildHelp, which has orphanages in many countries. The donations from the services support this charity.

So, with all that I have learned, seen, and witnessed in this life, I believe the world of healing is available to everyone. I now know for sure that we do not need to be healed at all. We accepted a mission to come to earth for this lifetime to learn and to teach. Some accomplish this from a wheelchair, some from the streets. Others with bodies that seem impossible or minds that continually challenge us are our teachers. Those who hurt others are also hurting due to lack of love. Those with chemical imbalances, malfunctioning blood chemistry, or poorly functioning parts inspire research with the help of technology. Leaving a sick body behind does not mean the soul is suffering at all. They are released, body free, a more educated soul than before. The traveling monks said that this earth provides all qualities of life. They said that in America, we have a roof over our heads and full bellies. Our karma was good. Give that some thought.

In Lak'ech.
You are another me.

CHAPTER

Eighteen

Demystifying Your Relationships Using Scientific Hand Analysis
By Michelyn Gjurasic

MICHELYN GJURASIC

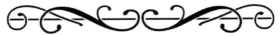

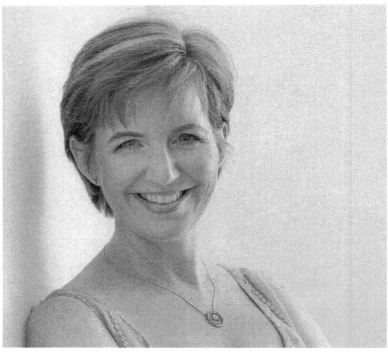

Michelyn Gjurasic is a Second Marriage Coach, because second marriages are different. She helps individuals, couples, and groups to navigate the three challenging phases of a second union: the "jitters" before the vows; the "oops" of complex compromises between two established families, careers and habits; and, the "double vision" of repeating patterns that are better left behind. Michelyn's passion is helping people feel successful in their relationships, no matter the label or the outcome. She is a Master Hand

Analyst and Certified Emotional Freedom Techniques Practitioner, as well as an artist, author, and speaker. She recently celebrated her 25th anniversary with her second husband. They live in Olympia, Washington, and have three children aged 22, 21, and 13. Michelyn works with clients both in-person and online. You can reach her at www.Michelyn.com, Michelyn.Gjurasic@gmail.com, or (360) 561-1591.

Acknowledgments

I'm not sure if I've learned more from watching bad relationships or good ones, but I'd like to thank the good ones for providing me with models to emulate. To Richard Unger, developer of the LifePrints system and my teacher, you have improved our planet with your wisdom and instruction. To Pamelah Landers, Empress of Permission and Expert Hand Analyst, my life has been immeasurably enriched by your powerful support. To my EFT Instructors, thank you for providing me with such a powerful tool for changing my life story and the stories of those I serve. To my best friends Lynda and Linnie, your steadfast love and laughter lift me higher every day. To my children, Alexis, Connor, and Kendall, thank you for letting me nurture you in the ways I know best. Now, go clean the kitchen. And to my husband Davor, for these 25 years together, I appreciate.

Demystifying Your Relationships Using Scientific Hand Analysis
By Michelyn Gjurasic

Painful Past

I watched the side door close from where I stood in the kitchen, dumbfounded. We'd recently gotten home from vacation, and my husband was leaving to "go to the store for a few groceries."

Yes, we needed the food. We'd been gone for four days, and the fridge was lean. But I'd mentioned stopping at Safeway on our way home to pick something up for dinner and to cover breakfast before I did a full shopping run tomorrow. He hadn't wanted to stop.

Now I watched him escape through the side door to do the same thing he hadn't wanted to do 20 minutes earlier. By himself. He obviously needed to get out, and I wondered what I had done to push him away. I felt confused, abandoned, and hurt after our wonderful long weekend of closeness.

This wasn't the first time I'd been left in the kitchen, watching my husband get away from me as fast as he could.

The Power of the Relationship Code

Fast forward one year.

I learned a few things after that day in the kitchen, the most important of which is that I am a Nurturer. The second most important thing I learned is that my husband is not. In fact, he's an Independent.

Nurturers and Independents are opposites in the emotional matrix. As a couple, we embody the full continuum from self-focused to other-focused, and from emotionally transparent to emotionally opaque.

Understanding these tensions has saved my marriage. Understanding your emotional style, as well as your partner's, children's, and co-workers', can revive and rejuvenate your relationships as well. The system I'm sharing here may be the most powerful game-changer you'll encounter for getting what you want and for feeling satisfied with your relationships.

The system is the Relationship Code. It's based on Richard Unger's LifePrints system founded in the early 1980s, which decodes personality and life meaning from the hands. I've studied and applied this system for seven years, and it has transformed all of my relationships, including my relationship with myself.

The Relationship Code focuses on one line in the hand, the heart line. To read yours, look closely at your palms. Most people have three major lines in each palm—two that start near each other on the thumb side of the palm and reach across and down, and one that starts on the pinkie side of the palm, closer to the fingers than the other two, that reaches across toward the pointer or middle finger.

Notice the shape of that uppermost major line—is it straight, or does it curve upward?

Then notice where it ends—under the pointer finger or under the middle finger?

If it's straight and short, ending under the middle finger without curving up to it, then you are an *Independent*, like my husband.

If your heart line is straight and long, ending under the pointer finger, then you are a *Thinker*.

If your heart line curves up toward the middle finger, then you are a *Passionate*.

If your heart line curves up but is longer and reaches toward the pointer finger, then you are a *Nurturer*. Welcome to my world.

Exceptions abound. You might be a Passionate on one hand and an Independent on the other. Your heart line might fork, giving you two, three, or all four different types, all on one hand. That's fine, only a little complicated. Having multiple heart line types allows you to connect with more types of people. You can also feel confused or a little crazy when you don't know which one to use or when. Knowing your types is the first step to feeling peace and clarity with multiple relating styles.

Now read about your heart line type(s) in the following charts. Odds are good you'll recognize yourself immediately.

While the heart line is one of the most significant markings on the hands, it is not the only one. Emotional styles are tempered by other factors. In fact, there are over 350 markings, shapes, and colors that make up the LifePrints system. However, there is much to be gained by understanding the four basic heart line styles.

The Independent

Qualities:

- Heroic, stoic, understated
- Reliable, predictable, loyal
- Work comes first
- Feelings percolate and process inside
- Shows feelings by doing

Descriptors:

- Element: Earth
- Needs: Freedom
- Likes: Control
- Hates: Clinginess
- Style: I'm busy
- Gift: Loyalty
- Common error: Shuts down emotions

The Thinker

Qualities:

- Thoughtful, considerate
- Feels lots, displays little
- Idealistic
- Subtlety and Nuance
- Spends lots of time in head—"Does okay truly mean okay?"

Descriptors:

- Element: Air

- Needs: Meaning
- Likes: Long talks, to ask why
- Hates: Conflict
- Style: Thoughtful, Considerate
- Gift: Romance, Idealism
- Common error: Over processes

The Passionate

Qualities:

- Fiery, intense
- Volatile, strong reactions
- Knows what she wants and wants it now
- Takes care of herself and expects you to do the same

Descriptors:

- Element: Fire
- Needs: Intensity
- Likes: Excitement
- Hates: Boredom
- Style: I want!
- Gift: Spontaneity, vivaciousness
- Common error: Acts like a Nurturer

The Nurturer

Qualities:

- Caring, giving, nurturing
- Feelings are close to the surface
- Empathetic, good listener
- Takes in wounded birds

- Likes to host Thanksgiving dinner

Descriptors

- Element: Water
- Needs: Connection
- Likes: Sharing
- Hates: Disconnect
- Style: Nurturing, Kind-hearted
- Gift: Sensitivity
- Common error: Gives herself away

Recognize yourself? Let's put some of this together in the form of an actual heart line analysis I conducted at a business fair a few months ago.

A Steamy Reading

Standing next to my display table with a handheld magnifying glass, I pore over the palms of a beautiful blond, as her curious husband stands by. I notice her slightly defensive posture, squeeze her hands gently and release them, then hold her eyes with mine.

"Your emotional style, your way of relating to others, has both water and fire energy. Many women with this heart line style emphasize the water side: they nurture, they caretake, they place others' needs above their needs. They're moms to everyone.

"They sometimes underemphasize their fiery, passionate side. Fire is spontaneous and exciting, but it can destroy whatever is in its path, leaving ashes in its wake.

"In our culture, girls are often told to 'be nice.' We're rewarded for being thoughtful and domestic. Being fiery and focused on our needs can seem selfish.

"Because of this, it's common for women with your heart lines to act like water and put their fire out. Can you relate to what I'm saying?"

Her stance had changed completely—her eyes were open wide, and her mouth hung open.

"Oh my gosh, how did you know that about me?" She exclaimed. "I hold back so much. It's like this secret I can't let out."

I nodded in understanding. "Honor your fire energy. It's part of you, part of your design, and ignoring it only leads to resentment and unhappiness. Understand that all the elements have both destructive and exalted potential. The key is to emphasize the positives and learn from the negatives.

"Your water energy can be wonderfully loving, conn- ecting, and nurturing. But water has a dark side as well—we can smother, dominate, and control those we care about. Inside, we can feel frustrated and burned out because we're overly focused on others.

"Conversely, fire can get a bad rap, but there's a positive side—fire exudes energy. It creates excitement and helps move things along. We are drawn to fire people as we are drawn to a campfire—for heat, for a spark, for action.

"The trick is to bring out your fire in ways that make you feel good while paying attention to your water needs. They're both in your hands, so they're both part of your design. You'll feel happier and more balanced when you can play with both water and fire."

Do's and Don'ts for Getting More of What You Want

The following chart is full of turbo-charged tips for navigating your relationships easily and getting more of what you want. Developed by my colleague Chrisstine Gulrajani, it's so practical you can put it to use right away.

The Independent

When interacting with me, please:

- Give me space
- Give me time to respond to your questions (maybe a day or a week)
- Know that I care even when I don't express my feelings
- Realize I love you even though I love work too
- Know I demonstrate my affection through practical actions

When interacting with me, please don't:

- Take my need for freedom personally
- Cling to me
- Be disappointed when I leave a party early without saying goodbye
- Betray me—I most likely won't give you a second chance

The Thinker

When interacting with me, please:

- Participate in conversation with me
- Appreciate my need for romance

- Join me in harmony
- Know I feel deeply even though I may not display it

When interacting with me, please don't:

- Ignore my need for conversation and understanding
- Pick fights with me
- Tell me that I'm over-processing or living out scenarios in my mind

The Passionate

When interacting with me, please:

- Realize I know what I want, and I will make it known
- Take care of your needs. I'm taking care of mine
- Give me time to vent
- Have a good time with me

When interacting with me, please don't:

- Spend time agonizing over an argument with me—I've moved on
- Be a wet blanket
- Plan when we're going to be intimate—be spontaneous!

The Nurturer

When interacting with me, please:

- Allow me to shower you with affection
- Create space for the injured cats I bring home
- Be kind when telling me I'm too clingy

- Gently encourage me to do something for me

When interacting with me, please don't:

- Disconnect from me without a reason or warning
- Stop me from giving to others
- Take advantage of my good nature

Now It's Your Turn

If you'd like your relationships to feel better, start with your relationship with yourself. Use the information contained in your hands, your unique design, to assess how well you are honoring your type.

- Here are a few questions to get the ball rolling.
- One of my heart lines is:
- This means that I like:
- And I dislike:
- Another of my heart lines is:
- This means that I like:
- And I dislike:
- My non-negotiable needs include:
- I can meet those needs by:
- Currently, I would estimate the amount of time I spend being my type at:
- Three examples of times when I have acted my type are:
- The times when I am not acting my type, I am being a:
- One current example of that is:
- Acting like a different type helps me to:

And Now, to Revolutionize Your Relationships

Ready to go one step further? Focus on a current relationship's trouble spot. If you can, take a look at that person's hands and identify their heart line type. If that's not an option, guess. Think about their behaviors—do they talk a lot or a little? Are they demonstrative or private? Do they need a lot of alone time, or are they the life of the party? See if you get a feel for their heart lines. Then complete the following sentences:

- I believe that my spouse/partner/child/parent/co-worker is a:
- This means that his/her primary need is for:
- And he/she dislikes:
- Our strengths together are:
- Our challenges together are:
- One thing I can do to improve our relationship is to:
- One thing I can request for myself is:

The Big Reveal

Now we get into the heavy lifting of the Relationship Code. Are you ready to go deep?

Think about a current relationship that is going well, that feels healthy and makes you feel good. Analyze the heart line styles involved and notice which characteristics were important in making the relationship positive for you.

Aim to get more of that.

Now ponder the past, and focus on a relationship that went sour. Maybe it started out gangbusters and fizzled fast, or it had a short honeymoon with a long, drawn-out downhill slide. Whatever happened, use your best guess to pinpoint the other person's heart line style. Draw conclusions using the information provided to find areas of conflict or disconnect.

Bonus Point Challenges:

Try these exercises for the ultimate stretch-and-grow:

Using the relationship-gone-bad example from the previous exercise, zero in on that person's most annoying, hurtful, and damaging behaviors and see if you can determine the motivation. For example, if he never gave you a straight answer to a straight question, and you conclude he was a Thinker, try that on for size. Thinkers love to talk about meaningful topics. For a long time. Giving a brief, direct answer to a question could be considered inconsiderate or even rude. You, however, if you're an Independent, value brevity and getting to the point, which leads to big miscommunication potential.

Next, try extending grace to the other person. Let some slack in the line. Pretend you're both aliens from different planets because one is a Nurturer and the other is a Passionate. You're aliens who meet up and decide to have a relationship. Step into their three-toed shoes.

Finally, communicate. Speak up using Relationship Code language, so you're not blaming anyone for being wrong. Let them know what's important to you. Ask for what you want and need. Recognize your non-negotiable needs, and theirs, and honor all of them. Show up for yourself, and you'll both feel better.

Congratulations! You've expanded your relationship

wisdom. Re-read this information until the Relationship Code becomes second nature to you. If you're anything like me, you'll find yourself watching people's hands as they talk at the coffee counter, in the classroom, and on TV. It's like having a secret superpower for quickly getting to the heart of what matters most in your relationships.

Painful Past, Revisited

Nowadays, when my husband and I come home from being away together, I do things differently. I know that for an Independent, being in close physical and emotional connection with anyone for a length of time can feel crowding. So I encourage him to take time alone to decompress. It doesn't lessen his love for me; it allows him to ration his close-up time with plenty of alone time so he can maintain his sense of self, balance, and freedom. Independents process emotions away from other people. It's better for him to do that with my blessing. Then I get the added bonus of being the one to encourage it.

Extending him that grace makes me feel generous and allows him his freedom. In return, because he knows this system too, he cuddles and listens when I need to vent. He'll hug me when I watch a sad movie, knowing nothing's wrong but understanding that I enjoy the catharsis of crying.

We're nimble with each other. We dance within the Relationship Code, depending on the rhythm of the moment. It's a beautiful dance.

CHAPTER

Nineteen

Healing Anxiety
Through Yoga
By Morgan Huff

MORGAN HUFF

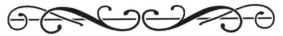

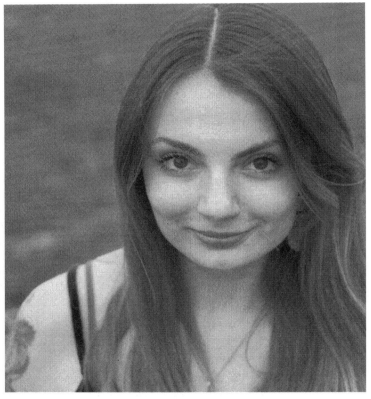

Morgan Huff is an Arizona-based yoga teacher. She leads empowered warriors suffering from anxiety towards their strongest self, on and off the yoga mat. Her passion is teaching trauma-mindful yoga classes for mental and physical resilience.

You can reach Morgan at www.morganasana.com. A final thank you to Kyra and Todd at As You Wish Publishing, and the teachers and students that have come before me to bring my journey into existence. Namaste.

Healing Anxiety Through Yoga
By Morgan Huff

D ear reader, I'm not going to start this chapter with a dramatic build-up, pumping undo steam into my experiences to tell you that I am the most qualified person to speak on the subject of healing anxiety. I can only speak from my healing and the testimonials of others. I am not a doctor, counselor, or licensed professional in any realm besides yoga. Even within this area, I can only speak from practices that worked for me over the last five years. What I am here to share is the knowledge I have gained—from my trauma and healing those traumas—and continue to acquire. Yoga has grown a confident, empowered, and resilient spirit within me that has grounded me in the path of sharing that life-giving knowledge and tools with you.

Perhaps you were drawn to this chapter as soon as you saw what I consider one of the biggest millennial "buzz-words" of pop culture psychology today—the word *anxiety*. Anxiety seems to be the big, bad wolf of mental health epidemics right now, often accompanied by its partner in crime—depression. One can only wonder why anxiety seems just now to be emerging as the hot topic in the mental health professions and pharmaceutical industry. Maybe it relates to the fact that anxiety wasn't a disease classified into the Diagnostic and Statistical Manual of Mental Disorders (DSM), until 1980. In the book's third edition, the formerly-known *anxiety neurosis* was split broadly between two categories—Generalized Anxiety Disorder (GAD) and Panic Disorder.

Those two 1980s, Grand Canyon-sized crater of categories don't begin to address the multitude of other anxiety disorders that we know exist today. Some of these include Post Traumatic Stress Disorder (PTSD), a slew of trigger-specific phobia disorders, as well as more acutely defined anxieties (e.g. "substance-induced anxiety"). I know, a shocker, right? Coming into a new age of psychology from one where previous medical ignorance suggested that people with schizophrenia be treated by the injection of malaria-infected blood in hopes the resulting fever would cure them of their symptoms—the same way that those suffering late stages of the sexually-transmitted disease syphilis appeared to be cured of a high fever. But thank God we have evolved since then, and new research allows us to learn more every day.

All psychology jargon aside, the following must be said because I feel it is important, when working with any kind of anxiety or trauma, to work with a licensed therapist or counselor that you trust. Then, once you know the root cause(s) of the anxieties you are dealing with, you can receive additional support from a professional. I cannot stress enough how important finding a therapist who creates a safe environment for healing can be. The best therapists help unearth and tackle the darker traumas of our past, which we might not have known we were carrying inside. Mental health is quite like sports in that if you want to win against the opponent (in this case, your anxiety), the best strategy is always from the offense, not the defense after the opponent has already launched an attack. This is the difference between being proactive versus reactive in supporting your mental wellness.

Let's Get Personal

Before I offer any further advice, I feel it only right to share a bit of my journey with that annoying inner-roommate we call anxiety, and how I found yoga as a source of deep healing.

Step back in time to 2014, where a 19-year-old Morgan has been lying in the Twin X-L bed of her Chicago dorm apartment, wearing the same sweatpants and Goodwill t-shirt for the last three days. Her eyes were nearly swollen shut from ragged, heaving sobs that seemed to start as suddenly as she thought they had stopped. She hasn't been to class in a week, has hardly kept down the Panera Bread broccoli cheddar soup that her concerned—and most likely frightened—roommate brought her in hopes of her keeping something down. The resident assistants have just knocked on the door and been wearily dismissed, after much reassurance that she was not suicidal or being harmed, but they have been alerted of constant wailing and signs of distress coming from room 2003.

When I say I was a wreck, I mean I was a *wreck*, you guys! The floodgates of hell had been unleashed, releasing the sparks of every stifled childhood tear and fear I was never allowed to fully process. Anxiety permeated my life after my previous highly co-dependent relationship had fallen apart. Its shadow fell on every corner of my daily life—to the point where I was afraid to leave my apartment. And what's worse is that I had been told by the boy from the aforementioned relationship, "You're not a nice person, Morgan," as the door hit me on the way out—after *he* had broken up with *me*. I honestly couldn't believe it at the time.

Now, I absolutely can believe it. What I couldn't see then, was that my anxiety had run my life and my choices for so long that it became a means of survival instilled in me since early childhood when my dad would rage at my mom or me, or she would flip into a seemingly manic episode. I wasn't validated to cry or hurt. I was supposed to suck it up and move on, expected to live in a cycle of unrealistically high standards. Performing became not only my art of surviving at home, but my escape from reality. The inner child in me found relief in theater and music—stepping out of my body and into someone else's. Call it artistic dissociation if you will!

Logically, it made sense that I ran toward that private art school in Chicago, which cost more than an exotic car in tuition each year, to pursue a degree in musical theatre performance. Boy, if you could have seen my dad's wrath and disappointment from his straight-A child getting her mom to co-sign for those loans without his permission. Even more disappointing, art school only taught me who I wasn't. And who I wasn't was someone made for multiple areas of perfection, constantly under scrutiny, with the looming pressure of money and adulthood survival—everything at stake from how many pirouettes I could do.

The young workaholic that I was, I added to my 18 credit-hour first semester: a part-time job at a workout studio doing princess parties, private voice lessons, and a work-study program at a dance studio—all so I could go right from my college dance class straight to three more hours of ballet.

Everything I did was in radical, clinging hope of one day achieving perfect, Broadway-worthy, "triple threat" status.

What I didn't know at the time was that I was one nervous breakdown away from completely changing the course of my life—for the better. And thank you sweet baby Jesus, for the day after the self-pity wallowing Morgan I mentioned above woke up and saw a flyer for a student recreation center yoga class. She ran to the nearest TJ Maxx and bought her first cheap, blue, no-grip-whatsoever yoga mat and headed to that class on Saturday morning. Since it was the weekend, there were no dance classes to be had or homework to be done as a distraction. And I needed endorphins—pronto.

I walked to my first yoga class—to the perfect ballerina-sized, toned body of my first yoga instructor, Dana. Dana had the looks and spirit of a fairy-godmother-pixie with a seemingly God-given hyper-flexibility and graceful strength that overtook every ounce of negative energy in the room. Everyone was completely focused on themselves, obliviously unaware of what any other person in the room was doing throughout the class. To this day, I'm unyieldingly grateful as I lie in savasana, or final resting pose. Lying flat on my back at the end of the class, an endless flood of silent tears and layers of emotional pain seemed to shed from my body, seeping into the mat beneath me.

Now, for anyone else who has never been to yoga—or maybe you went to one class and the teacher didn't resonate with you, or it seemed impossibly hard or uncomfortable for you—please lean into what I am about to say—that is where yoga works its magic. Right there, in the deep, fiery wrath of burning quads in a warrior pose; the deep opening of what seems like doomed, inflexible hip muscles during pigeon pose; the core work or arm balances you're told to "play" with—that look like a one-way ticket to the emergency room—with the weak chicken arms you wouldn't dare to attempt that kind of tomfoolery with!

I challenge you to ask yourself what might happen if, instead of judging or comparing yourself, you lean into the discomfort and emotions that come up in that moment. Greet each one with an observant, objective spirit, and ask yourself, what if?

What if I decided to accept being uncomfortable?

What if I look at what this is triggering for me emotionally?

What if I decided to rewrite the pattern?

What if I gave it my all for just another 5, 10, 30 seconds?

What if I decided not to leave the class and stay curious until the end?

What if I proved to myself that I *can* do this?

What if I fought for myself relentlessly for this hour?

Did any of those "what-ifs" resonate with you? Sit with it for a minute. Close your eyes, one hand on your heart and one hand on your belly, and breathe into a time where you wanted to rewrite the narrative later. What comes up for you?

Could you believe me if I told you that I have, and still do, battle with every one of those questions every time I step on my yoga mat—even now as a practitioner and teacher of five years? Most of our biggest insecurities and negative inner voices fueling anxiety and depression often sting with the undertone of shame. Even best-selling author and renowned therapist Brené Brown can agree, "Shame [is] the intensely painful feeling or experience of believing that we are flawed and therefore unworthy of love and belonging – something we've experienced, done, or failed to do makes us unworthy of connection."

In my experience working through trauma in a yoga practice, the single most effective ingredient to combatting shame is reminding myself of just how goddamn worthy and strong I am! Sometimes this looks like a sweaty, high-energy vinyasa practice, with space for adequate meditation at the end in savasana. The practice itself, being the moving meditation, moves nervous energy through me, harnessing it into renewed strength, and taking me beyond the pre-determined physical limits in my mindset before I began. Drop your shame at the door. Just move your body. Prove to yourself what a badass you are even if you feel weak. You are strong for pushing through because showing up again and again, not quitting on yourself when it gets hard—*that* is strength. *That* is resilience, my friend! *That* is what you are instilling into the grey matter of your brain. Every time you challenge yourself physically, it creates that same endurance in the mind.

How to Start Your Yoga Practice

Find a studio in your area, read reviews, and check out their website and class description page. I always recommend any type of "vinyasa" style class for getting the best sampling of what the practice can offer. My preferred style of vinyasa is the Ashtanga Yoga method, which also may appear as "Mysore style" on a schedule. Ashtanga yoga is a series of postures separated by a partial sun salutation—or "vinyasa"—intentionally designed with the whole body in mind. This is an excellent practice to start with because it instills the student with discipline of practicing six days a week while developing a relationship with a teacher they trust and feel safe with.

Additionally, it is a practice that a new student will learn a little bit at a time, adding on more each time the previous postures and sequence is committed to memory. The teacher offers hands-on assists and adjustments for proper alignment and safety in the postures, to further instill them in muscle memory. The best part of the Ashtanga yoga method is the fact that once you learn it, you begin to feel and measure your growth physically and mentally each time you practice since it's the same series. This offers a grounding, ritual aspect that one day, you will be able to practice anywhere on your own.

Go to the internet! If you are crowd-shy and want to try a class in the safety and privacy of your home before you step into the realm of studios and group classes, I highly recommend sampling a bunch of different 20-30 minute classes that are free on YouTube. Additionally, online yoga platforms almost always offer free one-month trials for their yoga classes. Below are some of my recommendations.

YouTube teachers: Jade Alectra, Morgan Tyler, Kino MacGregor, Liz Arch, and yours truly!

Online Yoga Platforms: www.oneoeight.com, www.omstars.com, www.glo.com, www.alomoves.com.

Start with ten minutes of meditation. Sounds simple right? Well, it may catch you by surprise, but the yoga asana practice itself, or movement portion of the practice, is actually designed as a moving meditation to prepare the body to sit comfortably in stillness for meditation or prayer at the end. This usually happens in a comfortable cross-legged position, sitting up straight with a tall spine, and eyes closed. For some people, this is an easier starting point than the physical practice. For others, the opposite is true—I, myself, find meditation a challenge. Therefore, I suggest getting started by just observing the breath for ten minutes a day. Here is a link to my favorite free meditation timer app to get you started: https://insighttimer.com.

My final suggestion is reaching out to one of your favorite yoga teachers either via social media, email, or their personal website when they post offerings for customized online courses, one-on-one Skype classes, private inst-ruction, workshops, retreats, and trainings.

My sincerest hope is that this chapter has resonated with at least one reader out there who may also be struggling with anxiety and a persistent desire to live a more abundant, peaceful life. If that happens to be you, then I am fulfilled in the quiet knowledge that this chapter served as a tool to start your journey and lead you to the best resources available. Thank you for reading and cracking open the spine of this book to start your journey of healing in the first place.

"When we heal ourselves, we heal the world." Mark Nepo

Always remember: you are enough, right now, as you are…and you are worth everything.

CHAPTER

Twenty

How A Femoral Artery Tear Fueled A Career In Healthcare
By Traci Schmidt

TRACI SCHMIDT

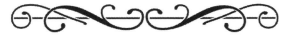

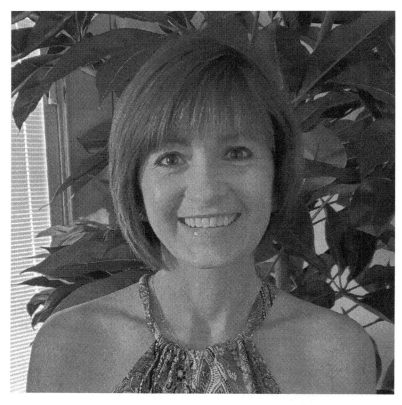

Traci Schmidt is a certified Institute of Integrative Nutrition health coach and survivor of severe environmental toxin overload. She is a mentor and health coach, assisting others with chronic health challenges to regain their vitality and quality of life. She is also trained through Precision Nutrition, Revolution in Motion, Electrons+, and other holistic modalities to help guide the body into healing itself. You can reach Traci at YourVitalityAZ@gmail.com.

Acknowledgments

An eternity of gratitude for my two boys who lived through my battle with severe toxin overload from childhood schools that were built on an industrial landfill. My boys were my motivation to fight for my life—and I won! My oldest son is a naturopathic doctor, and my other son is halfway through medical school. The passion to heal is within us!

How A Femoral Artery Tear Fueled A Career In Healthcare By Traci Schmidt

This particular case is about my son, Matt. Matt is a strong, young, and healthy 22-year-old who played college hockey for Northern Arizona University. During the first period of a late-night game, he was struck on the ice by an opposing player with what is known in hockey as a *knee-on-knee impact*. The pain was severe, but he stayed and sat on the bench as the game played on without him. After the game, he called me in excruciating pain, explaining what happened. He didn't want to go to the hospital, and of course, he wanted me to wait until the next morning to drive the two hours to take him to the doctor. He thought it was only a bad bruise.

The next morning, he was able to put a little weight on the leg, so he told me to take my time getting there. But within an hour, he called again, saying the pain was excruciating and to hurry up. When I got to him, his right leg was twice the size of the other leg, from his hip to his toes. I rushed him to the hospital, only to sit and wait while other non-emergency cases were taken ahead of us. His leg was turning cold in spots, and a golf ball-sized lump by his knee was pulsating wildly with his heartbeat. His condition was worsening.

Luckily, an orthopedic surgeon on his way home quickly ordered a pressure test on Matt's leg. Immediately upon receiving the results, he called for an operating room to be readied. The surgeon said he needed to release the pressure, and that the surgery would take about 15 minutes.

I sat alone in the surgery waiting room. After about 20 minutes, I was informed by the nurse that the surgery was going to take longer than expected. For the next 40 minutes, my mind was wondering what was happening to my son. My heart sank when the orthopedic surgeon came down the corridor. Something must have gone wrong.

He sat down across from me, leaned forward and rested his elbows on his legs. The fraction of a second before he spoke was almost unbearable. His first words indicated my son was still alive and had made it through the surgery, but that he had missed death by a thread. Matt had suffered a rupture to his femoral artery.

The surgeon replayed the surgery step-by-step. When he made the long lateral incision through Matt's thigh, the muscle actually popped out of his leg. He used his hands to show how he had held the muscle with one hand, then slid his other hand behind the muscle to scoop out a 500 cc blood clot, which then exposed the still hemorrhaging femoral artery. He explained that, because Matt's muscles were so swollen from playing in the game, it had actually helped put enough pressure on the ruptured artery to allow clotting to form. Had Matt decided to take an aspirin to ease the pain that night, his blood would have thinned and stopped the clotting, and he would have bled out and died. Or if he would have moved in such a way that shifted the clot, he would have also bled out and died. He was extremely lucky.

The surgeon explained that Matt suffered from a condition called Compartment Syndrome, and there was still a possibility of him losing his leg. Best case scenario, Matt was looking at multiple surgeries to remove necrotic tissue, or risk having permanent nerve damage or even having his leg amputated. My heart was broken for him.

He was in the hospital for three days. I wanted the best rehab/physical therapy possible for my son, so my thoughts instantly went to Dr. Simon Billingham in Scottsdale, Arizona. He was working with and developing a unique machine. I sent a picture with a description of the injury to Dr. Billingham and asked for his help. He told me to bring Matt in as soon as he was released from the hospital.

Matt was on crutches and could not bend his knee at all. Dr. Billingham, with his Electrons+ machine, guided a Pulsed Electromagnetic Field (PEMF) through his hands while testing Matt's muscle responses in his injured leg. There weren't any responses. Dr. Billingham explained that healthy muscles will twitch and contract, and unhealthy or injured muscles will not. Dr. Billingham used the Electrons+ machine and guided the PEMF into my son's leg for about an hour. He treated him twice a week for three weeks. By the end of the sixth treatment, my son was doing squats on that leg and had regained neurological function of his leg. My son continued to do the home physical therapy stretches and exercises that Dr. Billingham prescribed, and was back playing college hockey (against my wishes) for NAU by February of 2016, a mere four months after his traumatic injury.

Because of this incident, Matt decided to apply to Chiropractic School and is now in his third year.

What was this device that Dr. Billingham used?

Electrons+ is a form of Pulsed Electromagnetic Frequency (PEMF).

Much like a battery, the human body is electric. Our cells carry voltage. The electric charges necessary to maintain optimum health in our cells can decline from age, injuries, and illness. PEMF Therapy helps to restore this healthy electrical balance within the body.

Over the past 40 years, researchers all over the world have studied the effects of PEMF, conducting thousands of peer-reviewed studies. As a result, PEMF has been known for:

- Reducing, if not eliminating, joint discomfort
- Stimulating bone growth
- An adjunct to treat postoperative edema and pain
- An adjunct to cervical fusion surgery
- Depression in patients unresponsive to medications
- Reversing the bone loss and muscle degeneration

Accelerated Healing

PEMF treatments are known to accelerate the healing of any injuries, including wounds, joint pain, and tissue swelling. It is also used in the treatment of depression, allowing you to be healthier, stronger, and perform better.

Improved Pain Relief

Electrons+ treatment can reduce, if not eliminate, joint discomfort. It also feels amazing—like a supercharged massage. Your nervous system will be placed in a parasympathetic state (the rest and recovery state), which is essential for healing.

Proven Results

The beneficial effects of guided PEMF are often experienced after only one to three treatments. Some patients report immediate pain relief, improved range of motion, nervous system relaxation, and a general sense of well-being after the first treatment.

It felt like a miracle! Dr. Billingham, with the Electrons+, had taken my son's prognosis of a nonfunctioning leg or possible amputation to a full recovery with no deficits in his leg. The "unpreventable" necrosis and multiple surgeries to remove dead muscle never happened. Matt's cells, muscles, and nerves were given the proper energy to regenerate and heal. We are forever grateful!

Guided PEMF sends electrons into the cells, which are the rechargeable batteries of our body. Our bodies are comprised of trillions of cells, or rechargeable batteries. Groups of specific types of cells create organs, such as brain cells, liver cells, and muscle cells. Our cells are designed to function in a healthy manner at -20 mV (millivolts) to -25 mV. They replicate efficiently at -50 mV. So, when we are feeling fatigued, in pain, overstressed, recovering from an injury or surgery, our cellular voltage is low, and we need to be recharged. A healthy diet, proper hydration, and rest often are enough to recover from daily stresses.

"Chronic disease and loss of well-being is always defined by low electrical charge. With enough voltage and raw materials, the body can heal *almost* anything," (Jerry

Tennant, MD, *Healing is Voltage*). Dr. Tennant states, "The cells in the body are designed to run at -20 to -25 millivolts. To heal, we must achieve -50 millivolts," and "We experience chronic illness when voltage drops below -20 millivolts." And we experience cancer at +30 millivolts!

Electrons+ supports health by increasing microcirculation, sending electrons to your cells, which increases cellular activity, oxygen transport, nutrient uptake, hormone production, and immune cell function; thus, increasing your energy level, decreasing healing time, increasing immune function, reducing inflammation, decreasing pain, combatting chronic fatigue, and reducing chronic illness. Electrons+ restores cellular metabolism, decreases pathologic microorganisms that cause illness, improves lymphatic flow and drainage from inflamed and congested tissue, and recharges the cellular membranes, resulting in better cell membrane integrity and function.

The beauty and uniqueness of Electrons+ are that it is a guided PEMF, meaning the practitioner pinpoints the area in which the client is experiencing pain, inflammation, immobility, neuropathy, or lack of vitality. It is the only PEMF therapy available that is capable of assessing and determining where the blockages are. The practitioner, through his/her hands, guides the electromagnetic field therapy directly to the area of concern. Within one to three treatments, the affected area generally shows improvement.

I personally worked on a client who was a post-chemo/radiation patient that had the typical permanent residual effect of neuropathy of the extremities. He had 100 percent loss of feeling in one hand and 96 percent loss of feeling in the other hand. I started out working on his hands and his brachial plexus. After the first session, he had a tiny bit of sensation between his fingers when he rubbed them together—drove his wife nuts, because he came home wiggling his fingers nonstop. I worked on him again a week later for about an hour. I worked on him once a week for six weeks. He always said that about six hours after the session, he would feel the results. After session two, he started feeling the skin between his fingers, like he did before chemo/radiation, and experienced a tingling in the fingertips. After session three, the sensations were much stronger. By session six, he had 100 percent feeling in one and about 97 percent feeling in his other hand. He called me in tears after the sixth session because he had dropped a dime on his kitchen counter, and when he went to pick it up, he was able to pinch it between his fingers and pick it up. That miniscule task of feeling a dime or holding a pencil or feeling the keys of a keyboard had eluded him for three years. In six sessions, I was able to give him his hands back. He was an incredible artist before his cancer treatments. Since treating him, I have received multiple texts of pictures he has drawn, painted, airbrushed on canvas or scenes he has carved into antlers. My heart is filled with joy to know that I was able to give him his feeling, creativity, and a part of his life back. The last time I treated him was nine months ago, and he hasn't regressed at all since the last treatment.

Electrons+ providers around the country are having breakthrough results with some of the toughest cases in strokes, nerve damage, sports injuries, post-op, headaches, and chronic pain to name a few.

Electrons+ is being used by Rice University Sports Medicine Department, Major League Baseball, and the NFL, and more and more providers are adding this to their toolbox.

CHAPTER

Twenty - One

New Frontiers, New Discoveries And New Paradigms
By Dr. Vicki L. High

DR. VICKI L. HIGH

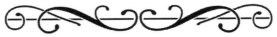

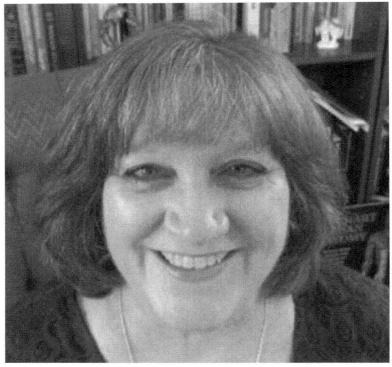

Dr. Vicki L. High is an international bestselling author. She has multiple best-selling books including, *Heart 2 Heart Connections: Miracles All Around Us*; *When I Rise, I Thrive*; *Healer*; *Life Coach and Inspirations*. She is the founder of Heart 2 Heart Healing, and is a Reiki Master Teacher, healing practitioner, life coach, counselor, speaker, minister, and former mayor. Dr. High, a pioneer in spiritual healing, boldly journeys into new frontiers of healing, love, and empowerment through spiritual insights. She shares intuitive and experiential wisdom, connecting ideas and concepts, and creating patterns for life and healing. She lives through her heart, honoring each person as an aspect of God–source. Vhigh4444@aol.com, www.heart2heartconnections.us, www.empowereddreams.com, @heart2heartprograms, @stoptraumadrama, @kalmingkids, @empowereddreams, @drvickilhigh

Acknowledgments

I am so grateful to my family and friends, the mentors and teachers in my life, and the spiritual family that has sustained me through so many adventures! Special thanks to Diane Sellers, Tina & Lon Morgan, Mom for the gift of laughter and loving family, H2H Practitioners who continue to spread their unconditional love throughout the world, fellow contributing authors, Kyra & Todd Schaefer, Janene, Jamie, Debbie, Darlene, and Ann for being great sounding boards. Thank you for your love and support!

New Frontiers, New Discoveries And New Paradigms
By Dr. Vicki L. High

T he leading edge of change brings new discoveries and new frontiers in holistic medicine. My journey into holistic healing began during recovery from a "surprise" divorce. For twenty years, I've witnessed miracles and seen lives transformed by new paradigms. As a seeker and observer, I love learning! Holistic medicine is an amazing frontier full of potential. This chapter shares my experiences that led me to explore these new frontiers, discoveries, and paradigms.

What are alternative approaches? How can they help? Which one is right for you? What results can you expect? Let's begin by learning about them.

Heart 2 Heart Healing

Heart 2 Heart Healing (H2H) is powered by unconditional love. It has the intelligence of God, and taps into source without religious rules, beliefs, restrictions, limitations, or boundaries. H2H brings the greatest power in the Universe to bear on situations, illnesses, and injuries, while healing issues that impact our physical, emotional, mental, and spiritual selves.

Workshops attract people on their spiritual journeys to expand what they've learned in their faith and other healing modalities. People experience their spiritual gifts, and through that knowledge and the power of unconditional love, they develop those gifts. Just as your muscles flex when you work out, your spiritual muscles flex, and you grow stronger when exercising them.

I founded H2H when I was told that I was doing neither Reiki nor Reconnective Healing. When invited to call it something else, I did. H2H began as a healing modality, but its innate intelligence began to teach me. My mind began to process information faster, often reading a single page of information at a glance. It felt like my memory was upgraded to accommodate and access data easily, and that surprised me! My thirst for knowledge led me to create a spiritual library. One of my gifts uses the words I read to fill gaps or make connections to thoughts or concepts from totally different origins and sources. How amazing it feels to read a passage in a book and *know* where that puzzle piece belongs in the bigger picture!

In sessions, people began to speak, and the messages were fascinating. I first thought it was the client speaking, until I listened to the words that could only come from the ascended masters: Jesus, Mother Mary, Mary Magdalen, Enoch, St. Germain, Melchizedek, and the archangels, among others. One message from Jesus described it this way, "When I heal people, I heal them heart to heart." Another message announced, "Forget the Human Genome Project. Forget the NIH. What you are doing is healing DNA." In another message, I asked who was speaking. The answer? "The words are written in the sky: God, Jehovah, Akrazuel, Elohim—the names go on and on." I felt like I was being educated by the "Universe-ity!"

My clients reported meeting members of the Galactic Federation, experiencing string theory, and traveling in multiple dimensions. One client relived a past life as a soldier in vivid detail, while other clients reported a series of supernatural experiences, including God speaking to them in a voice they clearly understood. The masters, guides, and teachers only had one request of me: *lose my beliefs*. After some resistance, I realized I couldn't hear them clearly if I was filtering their messages through my religious beliefs. Information was coming directly from God, source, Universe—the ultimate authority in my life. I lost my beliefs. My eyewitness accounts of miracles from God began to break open those "belief boxes." As a scribe, I recorded the information and still read it often to inspire me, to love others unconditionally, and live what I learned. H2H started out as a healing modality, but became my spiritual practice and way of life.

Early on with Reiki and Reconnective Healing, I experienced consistent miracles. I *knew* that the power came through the sacred heart. This was not a lesson from either modality. The sacred heart was and still is the power center for H2H. It is like an umbilical cord connected directly to God. The more I provide H2H for others, the more my heart is opened, and the greater the flow of H2H.

H2H Healing Experiences

H2H Healing is conducted either in person or from a distance. It is a powerful catalyst for change and, although simple, can alleviate symptoms from injuries and illnesses. Here are a few examples of the experiences of clients who have benefitted from H2H.

A co-worker's husband was suffering from stomach cancer. After a single H2H Healing treatment, the doctor reported the stomach cancer was gone.

One client was diagnosed with COPD and a variety of illnesses that plague geriatric patients. She was sent home from the hospital to die. When I visited the next day, I provided H2H Healing. She began to thrive. You could see the difference in her vitality. She lived another eight years.

Another client diagnosed with Hepatitis C experienced one H2H session. The people waiting noticed she looked different after her treatment. When she visited her doctor, he seemed amazed at her condition. She was released from the doctor's care because there was no trace of the virus.

A client suffered from carpal tunnel syndrome and anticipated surgery. She elected to try H2H Healing first. The carpal tunnel was healed without surgery.

A baby girl was born with CRV, a respiratory ailment. After holding her and providing H2H for twenty minutes, she began breathing easier. Years later, when I checked on her, she hadn't experienced any other childhood illnesses.

H2H Healing Practitioners who volunteered at a local event worked on a mother with two autistic children. The mother was amazed as the children began to interact with the practitioners during and after the treatment. H2H helped this mother communicate with her children effectively.

One client's 80-year old mother was diagnosed with myeloma, described as cancerous plasma cells. This condition is similar to leukemia, but affects red blood cells. Because of her age, the client asked that I provide H2H

Healing. I provided seven distance healing sessions. The final prognosis from her doctors was that she was misdiagnosed. There was no sign of myeloma.

H2H Healing is effective with all kinds of injuries, illnesses, diseases, and conditions. These are only a few client experiences, but there are numerous others. What I have learned is that traditional or allopathic medical treatments include medications, surgery, and cauterization. H2H alleviates conditions without prescriptions, surgery, or cauterizations, although it doesn't interfere with them. There are times when allopathic treatments are needed, but a lot of the situations can be addressed through H2H without invasion of the body. If this is effective, and I've gathered evidence that it is, let's at least try these alternative approaches before we cut, burn, and medicate people who are already hurting.

Reiki

Reiki is not a religion, belief system, or dogma. Reiki complements and enhances the effectiveness of medical procedures and other holistic therapies by supporting the body's natural healing ability. Reiki works on the cellular level, the blueprint, and alleviates the symptoms, restoring the body to wholeness.

As a Reiki Master Teacher, my personal experiences showed me the effectiveness of Reiki as a healing modality. In a 2002 message, I was told that "Reiki opened the door for me. Reiki. Reconnection. These two doors are gateways—mirror images."

Symbols shared in advanced workshops increase the power. Each Reiki session, workshop, or attunement I conducted led me to greater insights. The attunements brought engagement by Ascended Masters into the experience.

The purpose of attunement is to elevate participants to higher energetic levels. My first attunement was memorable. As I meditated in the energy, I became aware I could see in my peripheral vision the outline of a monk's brown hood— that I was wearing. In my final attunement in the series to become a Reiki Master Teacher, my Reiki Master said she saw a red lotus in my heart.

Reiki has changed since 1997 when I began my study. With Reiki, you need to ask permission to work on individuals. It was taught that the "bad energy" came out the feet, so avoid standing at the feet of the client. Reiki was taught as a verbal exchange of information, and although there were teaching materials, it was understood that it would dishonor the work if it were published in a book. Now there are many books and many different approaches.

My conclusion, based on observation and practical application, is this: Reiki is a healing modality that is founded in the duality of Planet Earth. It has good/bad, right/wrong, light/dark aspects which reflect duality. The energetic frequency is of the earth and duality. For me, the rules and limitations of duality changed when I received a message from Dr. Usui in 2015. He said, "Oh, beloved daughter, thank you for continuing my work. It is a gift for you to bring forth this work with higher energy vibration for those who are ready to move to higher levels. It is a milestone in Reiki. (Shanti). Thank you for letting me come."

Reconnective Healing

In June 2000, I took another step away from my traditional spirituality and moved into another world. My encounter with Jesus in the seminar was the most defining moment of my life. It opened me to a greater understanding of who I am and what my life purpose is. These incredible experiences were changing how I thought and acted in the world, and although, at the time, I thought I was doing Reconnective Healing, it was later that I realized and understood that it was more.

From November 2000-2003, I traveled both as an assistant and on the staff of Reconnective Healing. For several months, and again on September 10, 2001, during our trip from Houston to Dallas, Dr. Pearl attempted to recruit me. The next morning shocked the world as airplanes flew into the Twin Towers. It took me a couple of weeks, but I accepted his offer. I still had to conduct my civic duties as mayor one week each month while traveling throughout the country, guiding workshop participants to understand the processes. As staff, I made announcements and introduced Dr. Pearl as he took the stage. In February 2002, I resigned from his staff and resumed my duties as mayor.

My guides shared that Reconnective Healing was their way of bringing me up to speed. The results coming from the healing sessions were not experienced in the same way by other Reconnective Healing Practitioners. I know—I asked. I needed validation that I wasn't crazy, and at the same time, these experiences changed my life and me. Finally, a conversation with Dr. Pearl cleared the way for me to move forward in a new direction. He said, "Vicki, I don't know what you're doing. Call it something else." He did invite me to continue my relationship with Reconnective Healing, which I did until November 2003.

Although I continued to assist in seminars, I learned some valuable lessons about the healing community. The vast majority I met treated me with love and respect. Some remained steadfast friends. Others treated me like a leper. Still others seemed afraid they might fall from grace by association. No one wanted to be booted from the inner circle. I was hurt by false accusations and confused that a spiritual community could treat people callously. Eventually, I chalked it up to spiritual lessons, and knew I was stronger because I survived it, learned from it, and grew empowered by it. As spiritual seekers, we must walk our talk.

Psychic Surgery

I knew absolutely nothing about psychic surgery until I volunteered to help organize appointments for clients at the event. My first impression of Reverend Romy and his wife was that they looked much younger than I expected. They devoutly read their Bibles, quietly interacted with us, and then proceeded to do miraculous things with their hands, Tiger Balm, and a Styrofoam bowl.

For years, I experienced trouble with fibroid tumors. Reverend Romy removed them without tools, using only his hands. A friend who was in the room said, "I saw him remove those tumors from your uterus!" While working, he asked me to recite the Lord's Prayer. I know it like I know my name, but I couldn't remember a single word, so I kept repeating, "Adonai." I could feel pressure, and then it was finished. On another occasion, he took what looked like a cotton plug closely resembling a piece of razor clam from my third eye. I can't explain it, but that's what happened.

I read accusations saying that, allegedly, animal parts from the grocery store were used. I was with this lovely couple 24 hours each day. They never went anywhere they could purchase those things. One day while they went to lunch, I stayed and looked in every cabinet. I found nothing.

One day, Reverend Romy asked if I would assist him. I was so excited and agreed immediately. I watched as he removed tumors. He would run his finger down the area, a small amount of watery blood would appear along the "incision," and he would reach in and remove the tumor. My job was to "run energy," so I'd do H2H on the client, and then I would hold the bowl that would contain the tumor or tissue that had been removed. Reverend Romy had an extraordinary gift that helped people. He said, "One of these days people will not need to see what's removed." I knew at that moment he was describing the impact of H2H. H2H Healing happens without the physical incisions and tumor removal. My time with him was complete, but never forgotten.

Other Modalities

In my journey as a spiritual seeker, I became curious about other modalities. I allowed myself to explore when I felt an urge to learn. A friend invited me to learn Emo Trance, used to release tangled emotions. Matrix Energetics utilized a dashboard to change conditions in my life. EFT, or tapping, changed patterns. Acupressure and acupuncture relieved symptoms by clearing the meridians. Soul Recreation Therapy (SRT) was fascinating as it affected change by using a pendulum, charts, and Biblical references. Each modality has a purpose. Give yourself permission to explore and assuage your curiosity. Expand your horizons! The frontier of you can only be explored by you!

Conclusion

Fear keeps us from exploring these new frontiers, discoveries, and paradigms. Often that seed of fear grows with Herculean attempts to pass laws that prevent access to natural, holistic healing. Who benefits from that? Often it is a fear of monetary loss that keeps the government, corporations, hospitals, and Big Pharma spending billions funding and influencing drug trials, contributing to political campaigns, and spreading fear of natural remedies. It's exciting to realize the time for us to stand and acknowledge the amazing benefits of holistic healing is now. It's time to alleviate fear and exercise our power, our voices, and our purposes to live extraordinary, holistic lives.

CHAPTER

Twenty-Two

Clear Your Past,
Heal Your Present
By YuSon Shin

281

YUSON SHIN

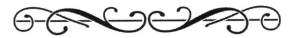

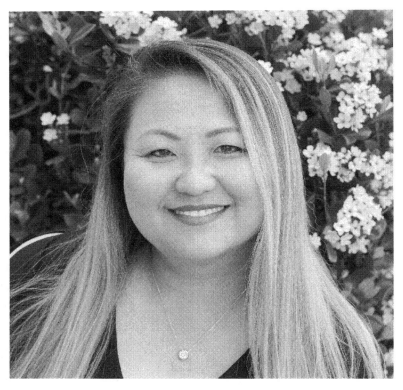

YuSon Shin is a healer, psychic, medium, and teacher of the healing and intuitive arts. She helps individuals heal themselves using past life, karma, and ancestral clearing techniques utilizing the Akashic records and Chinese energy healing. She is also a practitioner of the Bengston Energy Healing Method, Reiki (Usui, Archangel, and Kundalini), Integrated Energy Therapy, 5th Dimensional Quantum Healing, Quantum Touch, DNA Theta, and Access Bars. Her passion is teaching and helping people awaken their spiritual gifts and superpowers. You can reach YuSon at YuSon@ShinHealingArts.com, and get more information at www.ShinHealingArts.com.

Acknowledgments

I am eternally grateful to my amazing mother. She supports me without understanding what I do and does so out of unconditional love. A big thank you to Peanut, who waits patiently for me to finish my client sessions for her walks. A special thanks to all my teachers, students, clients, friends, and readers.

Clear Your Past, Heal Your Present
By YuSon Shin

Accessing My Inner Healer

I have always been a healer. However, I only became fully aware of this and recognized it in my 20s. Furthermore, being a late bloomer, I only started to embrace this aspect of myself in my 40s. Healing has always been a part of me though, and all my life, I have heard phrases such as, "You're a great listener," "I don't know why I'm telling you this," "You're so easy to talk to," "I feel better after spending time with you," "You have magic hands," or "My cat isn't friendly, but he likes you." Perhaps you have heard some of these phrases as well.

The biggest struggle I faced in becoming an energy healer was internal. Being left-brain dominant, I was raised to be logical, analytical, and require proof of all things unseen. I didn't purposely shut down my intuitive, creative, and emotional right brain. It was because my parents nurtured and only knew to reward the conventional, so I wasn't always a believer in energy and its impact. In fact, I was the biggest skeptic, and I thought that it was for airy-fairy people who did not have a firm grip on reality. Energy healing requires the ability to believe in and feel energy and its impact.

Synchronicities led me onto this healing path. I kept seeing these exact quotes by people I admired. Albert Einstein said, "The only real valuable thing is intuition." Steve Jobs of Apple, Inc. said, "Intuition is more powerful than intellect." Richard Branson of Virgin Group, Ltd. said, "I rely more on gut instinct than researching huge amounts of statistics." Being a practical person, I made the connection that tapping into my intuition would help me in my corporate career. On my journey, I discovered that my intuitive superpowers were the foundation for healing and life. The other powerful quality I unearthed about myself was my empathy. Without knowing how or why I could feel what others were feeling, I could share their pain, sadness, excitement, and happiness. And more importantly, I was able to gauge the temperament of my emotionally volatile father.

Energy and Its Relationship with Disease

Let's look at how disease occurs. Disease first shows up in a person's energy field. When that energy field isn't cleaned out, vibrations pertaining to that issue become increasingly absorbed, eventually materializing into an energy block. When there's a block or imbalance in the energy flow that's left unchecked, illness or disease soon occur. This can manifest physically, emotionally, mentally, spiritually, or financially. It's signaled in the form of high blood pressure, diabetes, IBS, depression, loneliness, loss of connection with our Source and ourselves, and simply being broke.

The prevention or cure is to be in the *flow*. The flow is having space to simply *be*, and it feels safe and open to infinite possibilities. Have you ever been driving in traffic and then experienced cars moving out of your lane, creating space for you so you can move freely and fast? That's what flow feels like. It feels good. And barring physical injury or accidents, one should be able to experience perfect health and perfect abundance.

Here are the main ways energy flow can be blocked:

1) Negative thoughts and emotional patterns;
2) Prolonged stress;
3) Unhealthy food;
4) Environmental toxins;
5) Trauma;
6) Negative patterns or trauma passed down from one generation to the next (ancestral issues); and,
7) Past life or karmic energy.

The first five items on the list are self-explanatory, so let's investigate the importance of ancestral and past-life events, because what you don't know can still affect you.

The Past Doesn't Always Stay in the Past

Ancestral blueprints exist in all of us. What happened to your grandmother or your grandmother's grandmother can still affect you. We are shaped by our experiences, but we are also influenced by events that occurred in earlier generations. These past events create ancestral blueprints, which are typically shaped by the trauma, grief, shame, guilt, hopelessness, and suffering that affect us unconsciously during our lifetime. Transgenerational themes are transferred from one generation to the next. Children of parents who are of a certain economic status tend to stay within the range of their parents or a little better. On a darker note, traumas tend to keep us from moving forward by keeping us in a prison of unconscious behavior, and they leave genetic imprints.

Rachel Yehuda of New York's Mount Sinai Hospital published a study which showed that trauma suffered by Holocaust survivors can trigger genetic changes in the DNA of their children. It showed that one person's life experience can affect subsequent generations. There can be a transmission of trauma through *epigenetic inheritance*. It was shown that trauma has the ability to change the genes associated with the regulation of stress hormones pre-conception. Her studies make one think about the origins of Jewish anxiety.

Studies of pregnant Dutch women during the "Hunger Winter" period from November 1944 to the spring of 1945, found that mothers who were malnourished during their first trimester had children who were more likely to have heart disease and higher rates of obesity as adults. The traumatic stress in the womb transferred to the children, grandchildren, and great-grandchildren.

Scientists at Emory University showed that one could also inherit a memory of trauma. They trained mice to fear the smell of cherry blossom by accompanying the smell with a small electric shock. The offspring of these mice had the same fear response to the smell of cherry blossom even though they had never encountered the smell before.

Author, Jacqueline Woodson, was on NPR in 2017, and raised the question of ancestral or genetic memory in the descendants of African slaves who crossed the Atlantic in slave ships under horrific conditions. Her interview raises questions of whether the prevalence of high blood pressure and fear of swimming in large bodies of water among African Americans may be an epigenetic response.

My grandparents and parents experienced Japanese occupation in Korea when food was in short supply, and even lost their identities as they were given Japanese names and required to learn and speak Japanese. Shortly thereafter, the Korean War took place, and many families lost members and suffered shell shock and food shortages. My parents both suffer from high blood pressure, and my mom has diabetes as well. I can't help but wonder if some part of their physical issues is an epigenetic response.

Traumas can lead to inherited depression and anxiety, even if families deal with it by denial or silence. Future generations can still feel its influence, even without overt acknowledgment. Author and psychotherapist, Anne Ancelin Schutzenberger, wrote the book, *The Ancestor Syndrome: Transgenerational Psychotherapy and the Hidden Links in the Family Tree.* In it, she describes a troubled patient who every Sunday went out looking for stones, collecting and breaking them, and also catching butterflies and gassing them in jars with cyanide before pinning them up. He later found there was a family secret about his grandfather that no one spoke about. His grandfather had been in a labor-camp-type prison, where he was forced to break rocks and was executed in a gas chamber. Truth generally finds a way to surface.

We are supercomputers that can be programmed, and programming is powerful. When we're young, our parents program us, which is why we typically become models of our parents later in life. The good news is we can reprogram ourselves for our sakes and that of our descendants.

Next, let's address past life or karmic influences. This is typically where unexplained issues are rooted. For example, someone might have a phobia, but can't pinpoint its origin in this lifetime. Or if someone experienced a stabbing to the left shoulder in another life, they may experience recurrent pain in that same shoulder in this life. Or if someone made a vow of poverty or chastity in a past life, they may feel that they can never get ahead financially or romantically in this life. Or if one's mother rejected them in one life, they may have a terrible fear of abandonment this time around.

This affects us as we can be triggered by things in this life that we cannot explain. And we can also be drawn to things or people that are not good for us. How many can admit to dating the same type of person? We also can find ourselves trapped in behavior cycles and self-sabotage until we learn our lesson. Understanding our past lives helps us understand our motivations, desires, and current life challenges.

Healing isn't the only upside to resolving past lives or karma. Talents and abilities from past lives can be harnessed. For example, a foreign language can be picked up easily if the person lived speaking that language in a previous life. Or someone who was an engineer or mechanic in a past life can now fix anything. People who have never painted can paint like a master. Someone who has never had a lesson can pick up a guitar and play like a pro. It makes you wonder if past-life gifts help create child prodigies. But it's also important to note that these gifts can be tapped into at any age.

Healing Steps

By acknowledging and extending forgiveness to our past selves, our current self can experience growth and release mental and emotional symptoms like stress, anxiety, and fear. Edgar Cayce, famous psychic and medical intuitive, used past-life information from the Akashic records to diagnose medical conditions and healing would follow.

The most famous contemporary author of past lives is Dr. Brian Weiss, who wrote *Many Lives, Many Masters* and *Miracles Happen*. He has a daughter named Amy Weiss who developed cataracts at 25. She details on Oprah's Super Soul Sunday that she had tried past-life regression previously and nothing happened. But in one instance, her dad was giving a workshop at her place of work, so she went. During that session, she discovered that in her past life, she was an old man in the Middle Ages. Townspeople thought the hermit was an evil wizard and burned everything he owned. The fire burned his eyes, and when prompted for a lesson in that life, she heard, "Sadness clouds the eyes." After that session, her cataracts disappeared.

I, too, have experienced the healing and freedom that resulted from looking at my past lives. I am a healer, but when I started out years ago, I could not shake a deep-seated fear of persecution for being a healer. I used my intuition (regression isn't always necessary), and as I played my mind movie, I discovered that in the 18th century, I had to lock all my windows and doors and hide my family in the dark whenever anyone came knocking. I knew that the townspeople feared my ability to heal and predict the future.

Ultimately, my then-husband and I were killed for who I was. This gripping fear that once prevented me from fully stepping into my power dissolved when I acknowledged the events of the past and forgave my killers.

One of the most incredible healing sessions I facilitated was with a woman who experienced pain whenever she ate. She had seen doctors who ran test after test and could not find a reason for her pain. I did some hands-on healing using the Bengston Energy Healing Method, and also accessed her past and past lives. I saw that as a child and in her past life, she experienced child abuse in a basement. Simply by bringing up those memories and clearing them with intention, the pain went away permanently after one session.

Ancestral and past-life influences, both good and bad, should be acknowledged. That is the first step to healing and living our best life now. There is an old saying, "The truth will set you free." We can heal ourselves by acknowledging our past and its current effects on us, whether it is with blocks, limiting beliefs, negative patterns, or fears. By bringing them to consciousness from the subconscious, acknowledging the issue, forgiving ourselves and others, and having gratitude for our lessons and gifts, we can experience healing.

It doesn't matter the technique you use to consider and resolve issues. Whether it's the Akashic records or Chinese energy healing or past life regression, the trick is to approach all things with neutrality or detachedness, because we don't see straight when we are triggered. And once we clear issues, we can make our lives easier. Clearing energy blocks is like cutting away dead weight so that you can soar and enjoy optimum health, prosperity, career advancement, great relationships, and love. And finding your ancestral or past-life gifts is the ultimate present to yourself. With that said, I want to encourage you all to get friendly with your past.

Exercise:

1) Set aside some quiet time. Close your eyes and relax. Melt into your soul. Breathe.
2) Think of an issue, fear, behavioral cycle, or pain that is affecting you now and determine to discover the root cause. Decide to be ok with whatever comes up or if nothing happens. Be neutral.
3) If any feelings or images surface, look at them merely as an observer.
4) Release any negative emotions that bubble up like guilt, shame, greed, sadness, anger, and doubt.
5) Love yourself for your effort in this exercise. Love yourself for who you are. Love the lessons learned.
6) Re-write your story. Breathe. By doing so, you release the past and breathe life into the new you.

Final Thoughts From The Publisher

It has been a true honor to work with the authors in this and all our other incredible books. At As You Wish we help author get their message to the world.

Visit us at

www.asyouwishpublishing.com

We are always looking for new and seasoned authors to be part of our collaborative books as well as solo books.

If you would like to write your own book please reach out to Kyra Schaefer at kyra@asyouwishpublishing.com

Recently Released

Happy Thoughts Playbook

When I Rise, I Thrive

Healer: 22 Expert Healers Share Their Wisdom To Help You Transform

Life Coach: 22 Expert Coaches Help You Navigate Life Challenges To Achieve Your Goals

Inspirations: 101 Uplifting Stories For Daily Happiness

When Angels Speak: 22 Angel Practitioners Help You Connect With The Guidance Of The Angels

Upcoming Projects

Manifestations: 101 Uplifting Stories Of Bringing The Imagined Into Reality

Made in the USA
San Bernardino,
CA

57176200R00171